Hemodynamic Monitoring

made Incredibly Easy!

Fifth Edition

Clinical Editor

Rose Knapp, DNP, RN, ACNP-BC
Associate Graduate Professor/MSN Program Director
Acute Care Advanced Practice Nurse Practitioner
Marjorie K. Unterberg School of Nursing and Health Studies
Monmouth University
West Long Branch, New Jersey

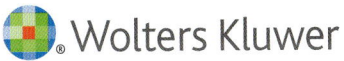

. Wolters Kluwer

Philadelphia • Baltimore • New York • London
Buenos Aires • Hong Kong • Sydney • Tokyo

Vice President and Segment Leader, Health Learning & Practice: Julie K. Stegman
Director, Nursing Education and Practice Content: Jamie Blum
Senior Acquisitions Editor: Joyce Berendes
Senior Development Editor: Meredith L. Brittain
Editorial Coordinator: Varshaanaa SM
Marketing Manager: Amy Whitaker
Editorial Assistant: Sara Thul
Manager, Graphic Arts and Design: Stephen Druding
Art Director, Illustration: Jennifer Clements
Production Project Manager: Kirstin Johnson
Manufacturing Coordinator: Bernard Tomboc
Prepress Vendor: S4Carlisle Publishing Services

Fifth Edition

Copyright © 2025 Wolters Kluwer.

Copyright © 2020 Wolters Kluwer. Copyright © 2015, 2010, 1990. All rights reserved. This book is protected by copyright. No part of this book may be reproduced or transmitted in any form or by any means, including as photocopies or scanned-in or other electronic copies, or utilized by any information storage and retrieval system without written permission from the copyright owner, except for brief quotations embodied in critical articles and reviews. Materials appearing in this book prepared by individuals as part of their official duties as U.S. government employees are not covered by the above-mentioned copyright. To request permission, please contact Wolters Kluwer at Two Commerce Square, 2001 Market Street, Philadelphia, PA 19103, via email at permissions@lww.com, or via our website at shop.lww.com (products and services).

9 8 7 6 5 4 3 2 1

Printed in Mexico

Library of Congress Cataloging-in-Publication Data

ISBN-13: 978-1-975235-95-6
ISBN-10: 1-975235-95-9

Library of Congress Control Number: 2024913386

This work is provided "as is," and the publisher disclaims any and all warranties, express or implied, including any warranties as to accuracy, comprehensiveness, or currency of the content of this work.

This work is no substitute for individual patient assessment based upon healthcare professionals' examination of each patient and consideration of, among other things, age, weight, gender, current or prior medical conditions, medication history, laboratory data and other factors unique to the patient. The publisher does not provide medical advice or guidance and this work is merely a reference tool. Healthcare professionals, and not the publisher, are solely responsible for the use of this work including all medical judgments and for any resulting diagnosis and treatments.

Given continuous, rapid advances in medical science and health information, independent professional verification of medical diagnoses, indications, appropriate pharmaceutical selections and dosages, and treatment options should be made and healthcare professionals should consult a variety of sources. When prescribing medication, healthcare professionals are advised to consult the product information sheet (the manufacturer's package insert) accompanying each drug to verify, among other things, conditions of use, warnings and side effects and identify any changes in dosage schedule or contraindications, particularly if the medication to be administered is new, infrequently used or has a narrow therapeutic range. To the maximum extent permitted under applicable law, no responsibility is assumed by the publisher for any injury and/or damage to persons or property, as a matter of products liability, negligence law or otherwise, or from any reference to or use by any person of this work.

shop.lww.com

QUADM0924

Dedication

To all critical care nurses who weathered incredible professional and personal challenges during our recent pandemic: May the content in this text be helpful as you meet the challenges of caring for the critically ill.

To my mentors, colleagues, and family: Thank you for your continued support and encouragement.

Rose Knapp, DNP, RN, ACNP-BC

Contributors

Susan Barnason, PhD, RN, APRN-CNS, CCRN, CEN, FAEN, FAHA, FAAN
Christine Heide Sorensen Endowed
  Professor of Nursing
University of NE Medical Center
College of Nursing
Lincoln, Nebraska

Natalie Burkhalter, MSN, CNS, FNP, ACNP, APN-BC
Consultant for Mercy Ministries of Laredo
Laredo, Texas

Sally Dye, DNP, APRN, ACNP-BC
Cardiology Nurse Practitioner
UT Southwestern
Dallas, Texas

Nancy Elman, RN, MSN, CCRN, CHFN, NP-C
Heart Failure Nurse Practitioner
Valley Health System
Ridgewood, New Jersey

Julene (Julie) B. Kruithof, MSN, RN, CCRN-K
Adult Critical Care Nurse Educator
Corewell Health
Grand Rapids, Michigan

Tricia Marceante, RN, MSN, APN-C (Retired)
Nurse Practitioner (APN)
Gloria Saker Woman's Heart Program
CentraState Medical Center
Freehold, New Jersey

Kimberly Reda, RN, MSN, FNP-BC, CCRN
Monmouth Cardiology Associates
Eatontown, New Jersey

Anna Remy, MSN, CRNP
Acute Care Nurse Practitioner
Heart and Vascular ICU
Hospital of the University of Pennsylvania
Philadelphia, Pennsylvania

Michelle D. Staggs, APRN, MNSc, ACNP-BC, CCRN, CEN
Acute Care Nurse Practitioner and Nurse
Assistant Director of Nursing
The Orthopedic and Spine Hospital
University of Arkansas for Medical
  Sciences
Little Rock, Arkansas

Patricia Walters, RN, MSN, APN, CCRN
Sock/pVAD Coordinator
Hackensack University Medical Center
Hackensack Meridian Health
Edison, New Jersey

Acknowledgments

To my colleagues who shared their expertise in cardiovascular nursing for this text: Susan Barnason, Natalie Burkhalter, Sally Dye, Nancy Ellman, Julie Kruithof, Tricia Marceante, Kimberly Reda, Anna Remy, Michelle Staggs, and Patricia Walters.

Rose Knapp, DNP, RN, ACNP-BC

Contents

Hemodynamic Monitoring

made Incredibly *Easy!*

Fifth Edition

Chapter 1

Cardiopulmonary anatomy and physiology

Understanding the pulmonary system

The pulmonary system delivers oxygen (O_2) to the bloodstream and removes excess carbon dioxide (CO_2) from the body. *The delivery of O_2 to the cells is essential for cell survival.* The alveoli are the gas exchange units of the lungs. The lungs in a typical adult contain about 300 million alveoli.

A closer look at alveoli

Gas exchange occurs rapidly in the tiny, thin-membraned alveoli. Inside these air sacs, O_2 from inhaled air diffuses into the blood as carbon dioxide diffuses from the blood into the air and is exhaled. Macrophages are present in the alveoli and protect from bacterial invasion through phagocytosis.

Alveoli consist of type I and type II epithelial cells:
- Type I cells form the alveolar walls, through which gas exchange occurs.
- Type II cells produce surfactant, a lipid-type substance that coats the alveoli. During inspiration, the alveolar surfactant allows the alveoli to expand uniformly. During expiration, the surfactant prevents alveolar collapse. This illustration shows a cross-sectional view of an alveolus.

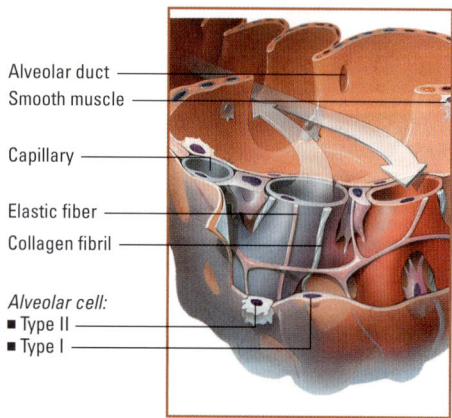

Alveolar duct
Smooth muscle
Capillary
Elastic fiber
Collagen fibril

Alveolar cell:
- Type II
- Type I

Structure of intrapulmonary airways

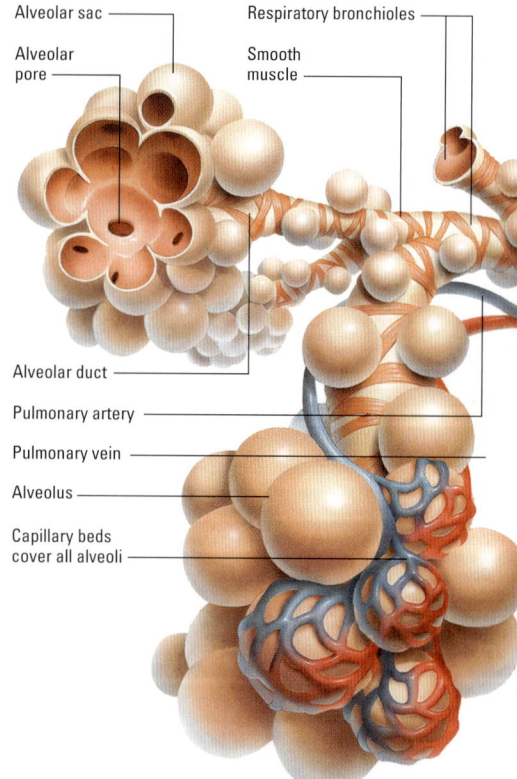

Alveolar sac
Alveolar pore
Respiratory bronchioles
Smooth muscle
Alveolar duct
Pulmonary artery
Pulmonary vein
Alveolus
Capillary beds cover all alveoli

Structures of the pulmonary system

The respiratory system is divided into the upper respiratory tract and the lower respiratory tract. The upper respiratory tract consists of the nose, mouth, nasopharynx, oropharynx, laryngopharynx, and larynx. The lower respiratory tract consists of the trachea, lungs, left and right mainstem bronchi, five secondary bronchi, and bronchioles. The left mainstem bronchus has two lobes, and the right mainstem bronchus has three lobes. Each lung is protected by a pleural membrane. The visceral pleura attaches to the outer surface of the lung, whereas the parietal pleura lines the inside of the thoracic cavity.

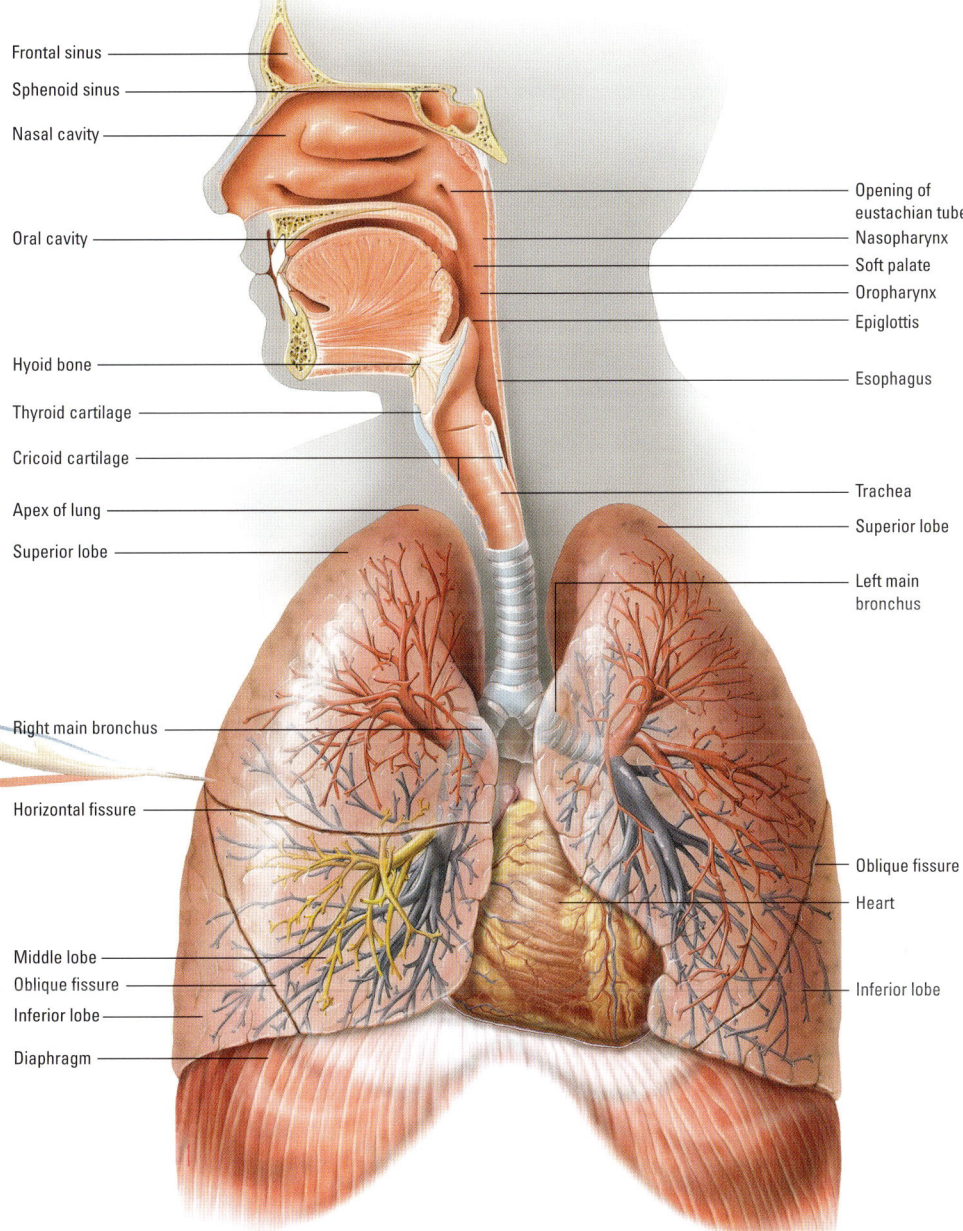

Frontal sinus

Sphenoid sinus

Nasal cavity

Oral cavity

Hyoid bone

Thyroid cartilage

Cricoid cartilage

Apex of lung

Superior lobe

Right main bronchus

Horizontal fissure

Middle lobe

Oblique fissure

Inferior lobe

Diaphragm

Opening of eustachian tube

Nasopharynx

Soft palate

Oropharynx

Epiglottis

Esophagus

Trachea

Superior lobe

Left main bronchus

Oblique fissure

Heart

Inferior lobe

Respiration

Effective respiration requires gas exchange in the lungs (external respiration) and in the tissues (internal respiration). Three external respiration processes are needed to maintain adequate oxygenation and acid-base balance:

1. **Ventilation** (gas distribution into and out of the pulmonary airways)
2. **Pulmonary perfusion** (blood flow from the right side of the heart, through the pulmonary circulation, and into the left side of the heart)
3. **Diffusion** (gas movement from an area of greater concentration to an area of lesser concentration through a semipermeable membrane): Deoxygenated blood enters the pulmonary capillaries, which have lower partial pressure of O_2 in inhaled alveolar air.

> Ventilation, pulmonary perfusion, and diffusion are the three processes for adequate oxygenation and acid-base balance.

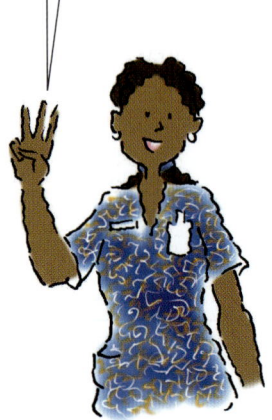

Ventilation

Breathing, or *ventilation*, is the movement of air into and out of the respiratory system. During inspiration, the diaphragm extends downward to allow a greater area for lung expansion. The external intercostal muscles contract, causing the rib cage to expand and the volume of the thoracic cavity to increase. Air then rushes in to equalize the pressure. The air moves throughout the respiratory tract down to the alveoli, where gas exchange takes place. During expiration, the lungs passively recoil as the diaphragm and intercostal muscles relax, pushing air out of the lungs. CO_2 is then expired.

The mechanics of breathing

Mechanical forces, such as movement of the diaphragm and intercostal muscles, drive the breathing process, which is a response to the changes in the atmospheric pressure within the alveoli and pleural cavity. In the figures that follow, a plus sign (+) indicates positive pressure, and a minus sign (−) indicates negative pressure.

At rest

- Inspiratory muscles relax.
- Atmospheric pressure is maintained in the tracheobronchial tree.
- Atmospheric pressure = pressure in the alveoli and lungs.
- No air movement occurs.

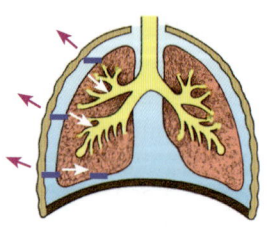

Inspiration

- Inspiratory muscles contract.
- The diaphragm descends.
- Negative alveolar pressure is maintained.

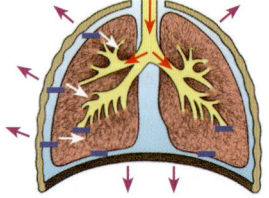

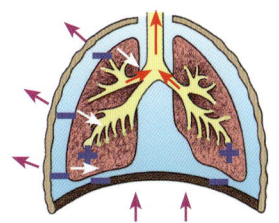

Expiration

- Inspiratory muscles relax, causing the lungs to recoil to their resting size and position.
- The diaphragm ascends.
- Positive alveolar pressure is maintained.

Pulmonary perfusion

Blood flow through the lungs is powered by the right ventricle. The right and left pulmonary arteries carry deoxygenated blood from the right ventricle to the lungs. These arteries divide to form distal branches called *arterioles,* which terminate as a concentrated capillary network in the alveoli and alveolar sac, where gas exchange occurs. After the deoxygenated blood flows from the right side of the heart through the pulmonary circulation, oxygenated blood is delivered to the left side of the heart.

Venules—the end branches of the pulmonary veins—collect oxygenated blood from the capillaries and transport it to larger vessels, which carry it to the pulmonary veins. The pulmonary veins enter the left side of the heart and distribute oxygenated blood throughout the body.

Tracking pulmonary perfusion

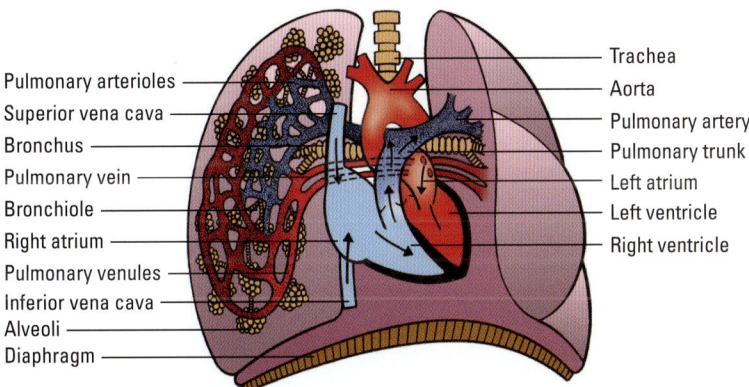

Pulmonary arterioles
Superior vena cava
Bronchus
Pulmonary vein
Bronchiole
Right atrium
Pulmonary venules
Inferior vena cava
Alveoli
Diaphragm

Trachea
Aorta
Pulmonary artery
Pulmonary trunk
Left atrium
Left ventricle
Right ventricle

Pulmonary vascular resistance

Pulmonary vascular resistance (PVR) refers to the resistance in the pulmonary vascular bed against which the right ventricle must eject blood. PVR is largely determined by the caliber and degree of tone of the pulmonary arteries, capillaries, and veins and is measured with the use of hemodynamic monitoring. Because these vessels are thin walled and highly elastic, PVR is normally very low. However, PVR may be easily influenced by vasoactive stimuli that dilate or constrict the pulmonary vessels or affect the tone of these vessels.

Factors that increase PVR include:
- vasoconstricting drugs
- hypoxemia
- acidemia
- hypercapnia
- atelectasis.

Factors that decrease PVR include:
- vasodilating drugs
- alkalemia
- hypocapnia
- conditions that result in high cardiac output, such as during strenuous exercise.

Diffusion

Blood in the pulmonary capillaries gains O_2 and loses CO_2 through the process of diffusion (gas exchange). In this process, O_2 and CO_2 move from an area of greater concentration to an area of lesser concentration through the pulmonary capillary, a semipermeable membrane.

Diffusion across the alveolar–capillary membrane

This illustration shows how the differences in gas concentration between blood in the pulmonary artery (deoxygenated blood from the right side of the heart) and alveolus make this process possible. Gas concentrations depicted in the pulmonary vein are the end result of gas exchange and represent the blood that is delivered to the left side of the heart and systemic circulation.

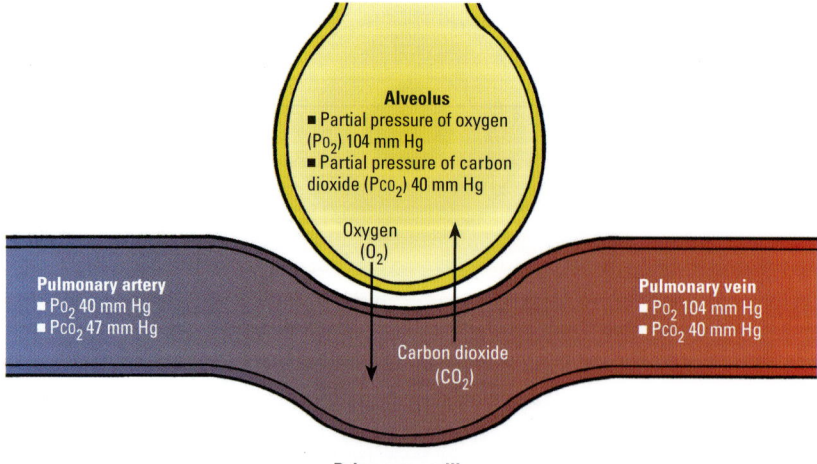

Alveolus
- Partial pressure of oxygen (Po_2) 104 mm Hg
- Partial pressure of carbon dioxide (Pco_2) 40 mm Hg

Oxygen (O_2)

Pulmonary artery
- Po_2 40 mm Hg
- Pco_2 47 mm Hg

Carbon dioxide (CO_2)

Pulmonary vein
- Po_2 104 mm Hg
- Pco_2 40 mm Hg

Pulmonary capillary

Ventilation and perfusion ratio

Areas where perfusion and ventilation are similar have a ventilation-perfusion match ($\dot{V}/\dot{Q}$ match). Gas exchange is most efficient in such areas. For example, in normal lung function, the alveoli receive air at a rate of about 4 L/min, whereas the capillaries supply blood to the alveoli at a rate of about 5 L/min, creating a $\dot{V}/\dot{Q}$ ratio of 4:5, or 0.8 (the normal range for a $\dot{V}/\dot{Q}$ ratio is from 0.8 to 1.2).

A $\dot{V}/\dot{Q}$ mismatch, resulting from ventilation-perfusion dysfunction or altered lung mechanics, indicates ineffective gas exchange between the alveoli and pulmonary capillaries and can affect all body systems by changing the amount of O_2 delivered to living cells.

Understanding ventilation and perfusion

When $\dot{V}/\dot{Q}$ matches, unoxygenated blood from the venous system returns to the right side of the heart through the pulmonary artery to the lungs, carrying CO_2. The arteries branch into the alveolar capillaries. Gas exchange takes place in the alveolar capillaries. This process is depicted in the below illustration, and possible causes of a $\dot{V}/\dot{Q}$ mismatch are described in the table that follows.

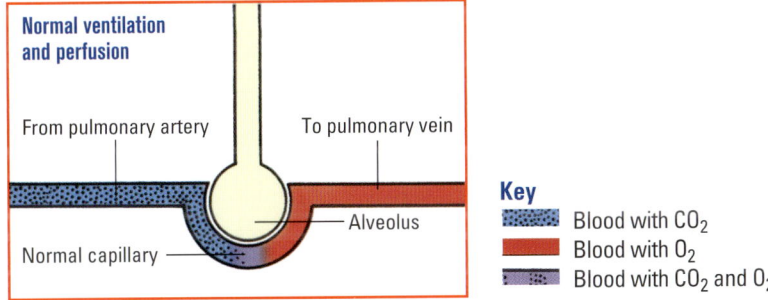

Normal ventilation and perfusion

From pulmonary artery   To pulmonary vein

Alveolus

Normal capillary

Key
- Blood with CO_2
- Blood with O_2
- Blood with CO_2 and O_2

Possible causes of a $\dot{V}/\dot{Q}$ mismatch

Cause	Description	Illustration	Explanation
Shunting	Reduced ventilation to a lung unit; perfusion is normal. Causes unoxygenated blood to move from the right side of the heart to the left side of the heart and into systemic circulation; it may result from physical defects or airway obstruction.	**Inadequate ventilation (shunt)** Ventilation blockage From pulmonary artery To pulmonary vein Alveolus	When the $\dot{V}/\dot{Q}$ ratio is low, pulmonary circulation is adequate, but not enough O_2 is available to the alveoli for normal diffusion. A portion of the blood flowing through the pulmonary vessels does not become oxygenated.

(*continued*)

Cause	Description	Illustration	Explanation
Dead space ventilation	Reduced perfusion to a lung unit; ventilation is normal; occurs but the alveoli do not have adequate blood supply for gas exchange to occur, such as with pulmonary emboli and pulmonary infarction.	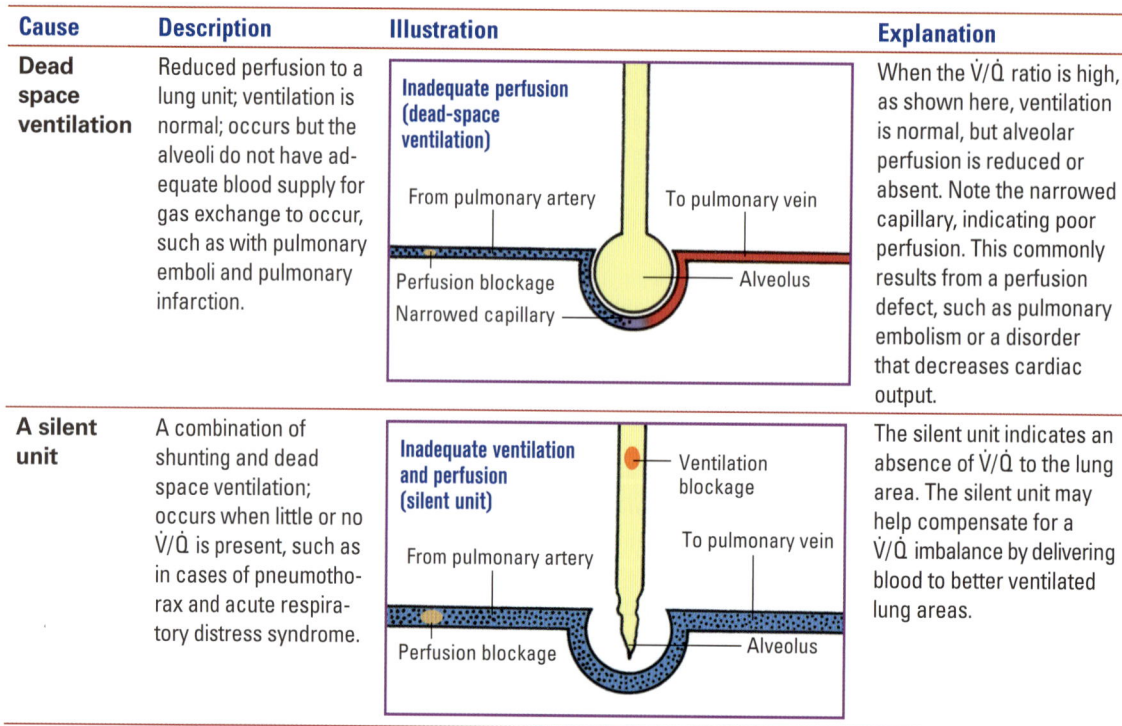 **Inadequate perfusion (dead-space ventilation)** From pulmonary artery — To pulmonary vein Perfusion blockage — Alveolus Narrowed capillary	When the $\dot{V}/\dot{Q}$ ratio is high, as shown here, ventilation is normal, but alveolar perfusion is reduced or absent. Note the narrowed capillary, indicating poor perfusion. This commonly results from a perfusion defect, such as pulmonary embolism or a disorder that decreases cardiac output.
A silent unit	A combination of shunting and dead space ventilation; occurs when little or no $\dot{V}/\dot{Q}$ is present, such as in cases of pneumothorax and acute respiratory distress syndrome.	**Inadequate ventilation and perfusion (silent unit)** Ventilation blockage To pulmonary vein From pulmonary artery Perfusion blockage — Alveolus	The silent unit indicates an absence of $\dot{V}/\dot{Q}$ to the lung area. The silent unit may help compensate for a $\dot{V}/\dot{Q}$ imbalance by delivering blood to better ventilated lung areas.

Understanding the cardiac system

The cardiac system:
- works in conjunction with the pulmonary system to carry life-sustaining O_2 and nutrients in the blood to all cells of the body.
- removes metabolic waste products in the blood from the cells.

   The heart is a cone-shaped muscle located within the mediastinum and is surrounded by a protective sac called the pericardium. The major blood vessels of the heart are the left and right coronary arteries, which branch from the base of the aorta. The heart is divided into four chambers: the right and left atria and the right and left ventricles. The right heart is responsible for delivering deoxygenated blood to the lungs and is a low-pressure system. The left heart is responsible for delivering oxygenated blood to the body and is a high-pressure system.

The valves of the heart facilitate the flow of blood in a forward direction. The atrioventricular (AV) valves are the tricuspid and mitral valves. The semilunar valves are the pulmonic and aortic valves. The tricuspid valve is located between the right atrium and the right ventricle. The mitral valve is located between the left atrium and the left ventricle. The pulmonic valve is located between the right ventricle and the pulmonary artery. The aortic valve is located between the left ventricle and the aorta.

A closer look at the heart

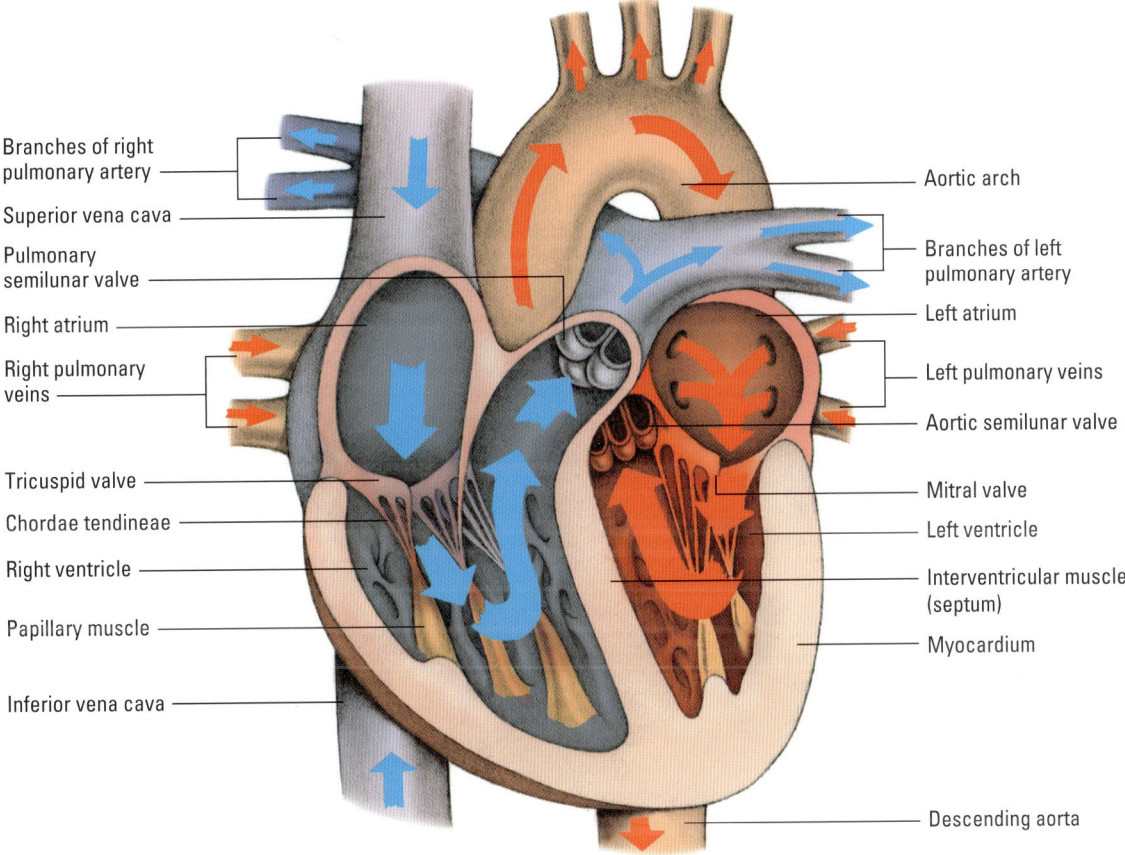

Branches of right pulmonary artery

Superior vena cava

Pulmonary semilunar valve

Right atrium

Right pulmonary veins

Tricuspid valve

Chordae tendineae

Right ventricle

Papillary muscle

Inferior vena cava

Aortic arch

Branches of left pulmonary artery

Left atrium

Left pulmonary veins

Aortic semilunar valve

Mitral valve

Left ventricle

Interventricular muscle (septum)

Myocardium

Descending aorta

Viewing coronary vessels
Anterior view

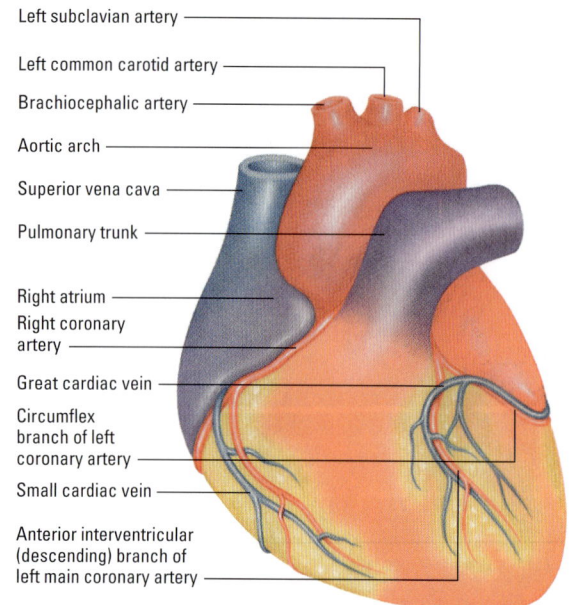

Left subclavian artery

Left common carotid artery

Brachiocephalic artery

Aortic arch

Superior vena cava

Pulmonary trunk

Right atrium

Right coronary artery

Great cardiac vein

Circumflex branch of left coronary artery

Small cardiac vein

Anterior interventricular (descending) branch of left main coronary artery

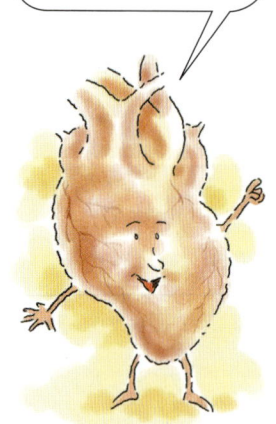

These two views of the heart might help you put together the pieces of the heart puzzle! They show the great vessels and some major coronary vessels.

Posterior view

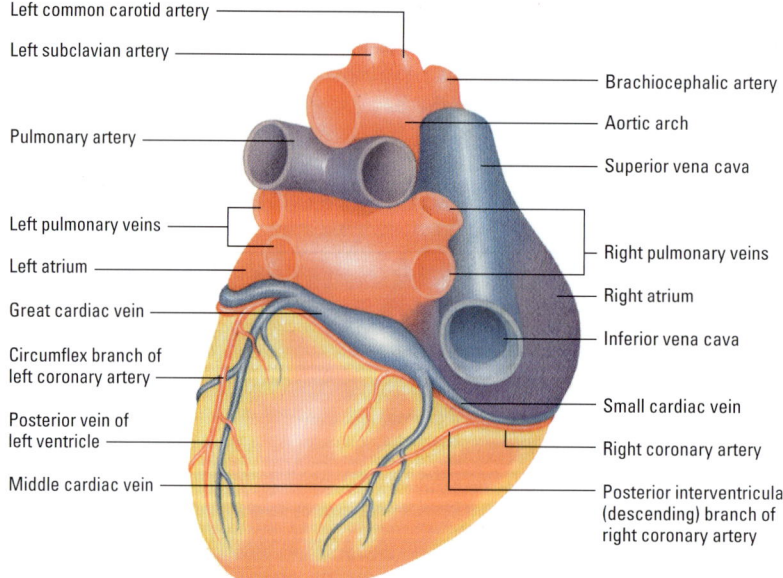

Left common carotid artery

Left subclavian artery

Pulmonary artery

Left pulmonary veins

Left atrium

Great cardiac vein

Circumflex branch of left coronary artery

Posterior vein of left ventricle

Middle cardiac vein

Brachiocephalic artery

Aortic arch

Superior vena cava

Right pulmonary veins

Right atrium

Inferior vena cava

Small cardiac vein

Right coronary artery

Posterior interventricular (descending) branch of right coronary artery

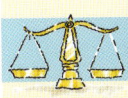

On the level

Normal intracardiac pressures

Structure	Normal pressure
Right atrium	0–8 mm Hg
Right ventricle	Systolic: 15–25 mm Hg
	Diastolic: 0–8 mm Hg
Pulmonary artery	Systolic: 15–25 mm Hg
	Diastolic: 8–15 mm Hg
Left atrium	4–12 mm Hg
Left ventricle	Systolic: 110–130 mm Hg
	Diastolic: 4–12 mm Hg
Aorta	Systolic: 110–130 mm Hg
	Diastolic: 70–80 mm Hg

Cardiac conduction

The conduction system of the heart begins with the heart's pacemaker, the sinoatrial (SA) node, which is located in the right atrium. When an impulse leaves the SA node, it travels through the atria along the Bachmann bundle and the internodal pathways on its way to the AV node and the ventricles. After the impulse passes through the AV node, it travels to the ventricles, first down the bundle of His, then along the bundle branches, and, lastly, down the Purkinje fibers.

Cardiac conduction system

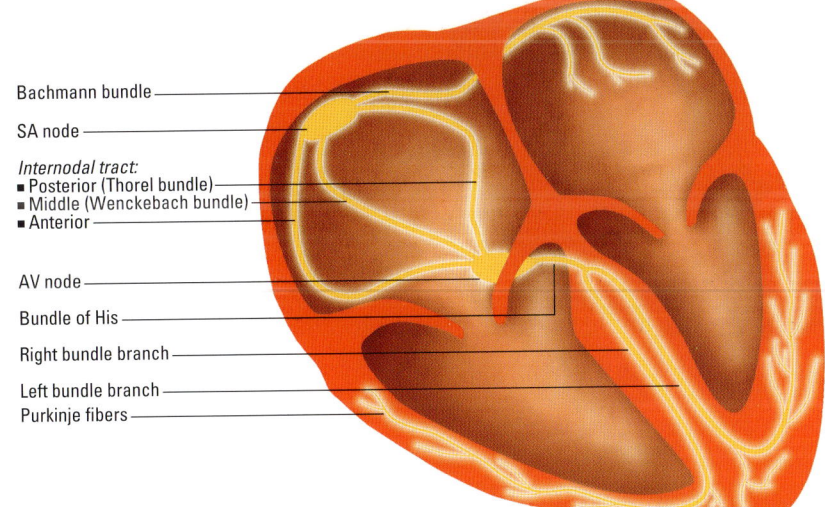

Bachmann bundle

SA node

Internodal tract:
- Posterior (Thorel bundle)
- Middle (Wenckebach bundle)
- Anterior

AV node

Bundle of His

Right bundle branch

Left bundle branch
Purkinje fibers

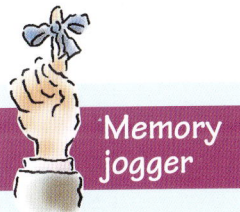

Memory jogger

To remember the path of cardiac conduction, use this mnemonic: **S**ome **B**elieve **I**n **A**cting **B**adly **B**efore **P**erforming.

The first letter of the words in the mnemonic stand for:
Sinoatrial node
Bachmann bundle
Internodal
    pathways
Atrioventricular
    node
Bundle of His
Bundle branches
Purkinje fibers

Events of the cardiac cycle

The steps in the cardiac cycle, described here, are illustrated in the figure that follows:

1. **Isovolumetric ventricular contraction:** In response to ventricular depolarization, tension in the ventricles increases. This rise in pressure within the ventricles leads to closure of the mitral and tricuspid valves. The pulmonic and aortic valves stay closed during the entire phase.

2. **Ventricular ejection:** When ventricular pressure exceeds aortic and pulmonary arterial pressure, the aortic and pulmonic valves open and the ventricles eject blood.

3. **Isovolumetric relaxation:** When ventricular pressure falls below the pressure in the aorta and pulmonary artery, the aortic and pulmonic valves close. All valves are closed during this phase. Atrial diastole occurs as blood fills the atria.

4. **Ventricular filling:** Atrial pressure exceeds ventricular pressure, which causes the mitral and tricuspid valves to open. Blood then flows passively into the ventricles. About 70% of ventricular filling takes place during this phase.

5. **Atrial systole:** Known as the *atrial kick*, atrial systole (coinciding with late ventricular diastole) supplies the ventricles with the remaining 30% of the blood for each heartbeat.

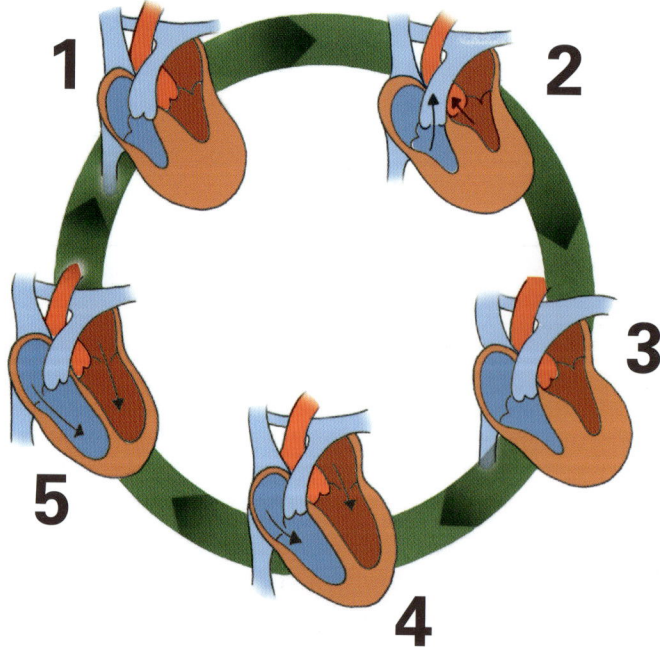

Cardiovascular circuit

The cardiovascular circuit is a continuous, closed, fluid-filled elastic system of arteries, capillaries, and veins. The heart acts as a pump for this system.

Blood circulation

Blood enters the right atrium from the vena cava and flows into the right ventricle during diastole. During systole, the heart muscles contract to send blood through the pulmonary trunk to the lungs for oxygenation. Blood returns to the left atrium through the pulmonary veins and flows into the left ventricle. Heart muscles contract again to drive blood through the aorta into the arterial system of the body. Because arteries become increasingly smaller, blood reaches capillary beds, where O_2 is released to the cells of organs and tissues. Veins then carry the O_2-poor blood back to the vena cava.

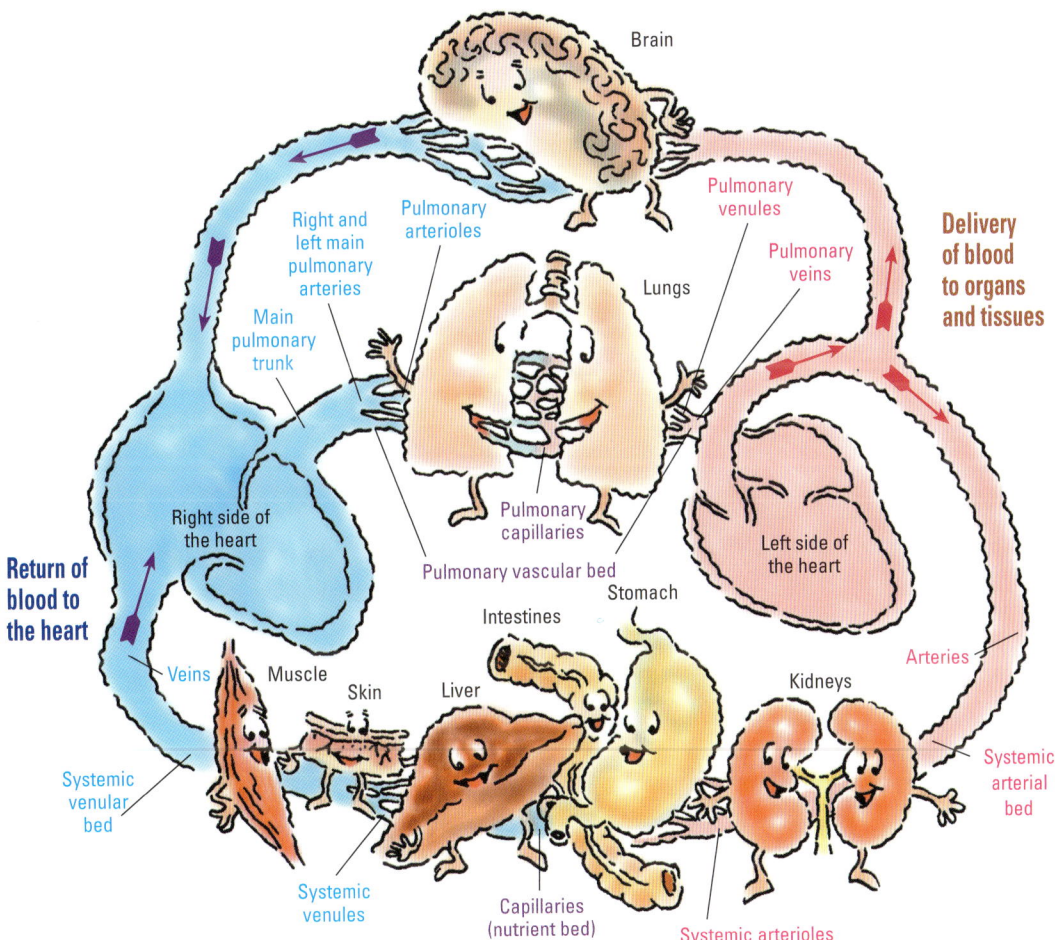

Systemic vascular resistance

Systemic vascular resistance (SVR) represents the resistance against which the left ventricle must pump to move blood throughout systemic circulation. SVR can be affected by:

- tone and diameter of the blood vessels
- viscosity of the blood
- resistance from the inner lining of the blood vessels.

SVR usually has an inverse relationship to cardiac output; that is, when SVR decreases, cardiac output increases, and when cardiac output decreases, SVR will increase.

Although newer electronic monitors can automatically calculate SVR from hemodynamic measurements, the following formula can be used to calculate it by hand:

$$SVR = \frac{\text{mean arterial pressure} - \text{central venous pressure}}{\text{cardiac output}} \times 80$$

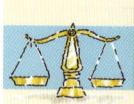

On the level

Measurements of systemic vascular resistance

Normal measurements of SVR range from 770 to 1,500 dynes/sec/cm^{-5}.

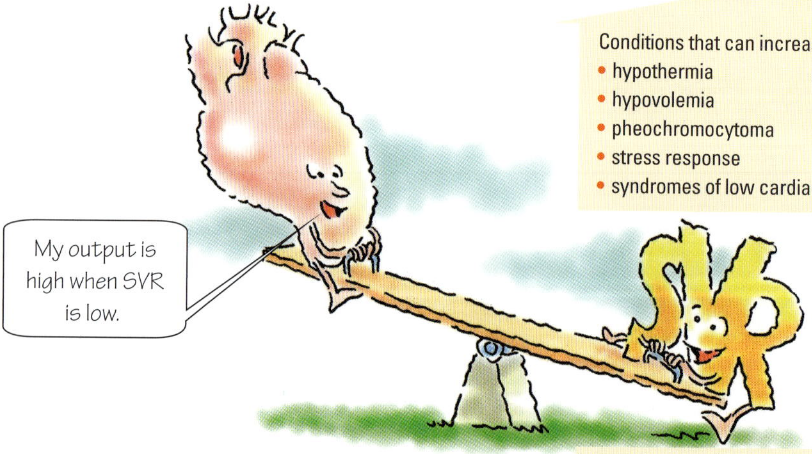

Conditions that can increase SVR include:
- hypothermia
- hypovolemia
- pheochromocytoma
- stress response
- syndromes of low cardiac output.

My output is high when SVR is low.

Conditions that can decrease SVR include:
- anaphylactic and neurogenic shock
- anemia
- cirrhosis
- vasodilation.

Cardiac output

Cardiac output is the amount of blood the heart pumps in 1 minute. It is equal to the heart rate multiplied by the stroke volume (the amount of blood ejected with each heartbeat).

$$\text{Cardiac output} = \text{heart rate} \times \text{stroke volume}$$

Stroke volume depends on three major factors:
- preload
- contractility
- afterload.

Influences on stroke volume and cardiac output

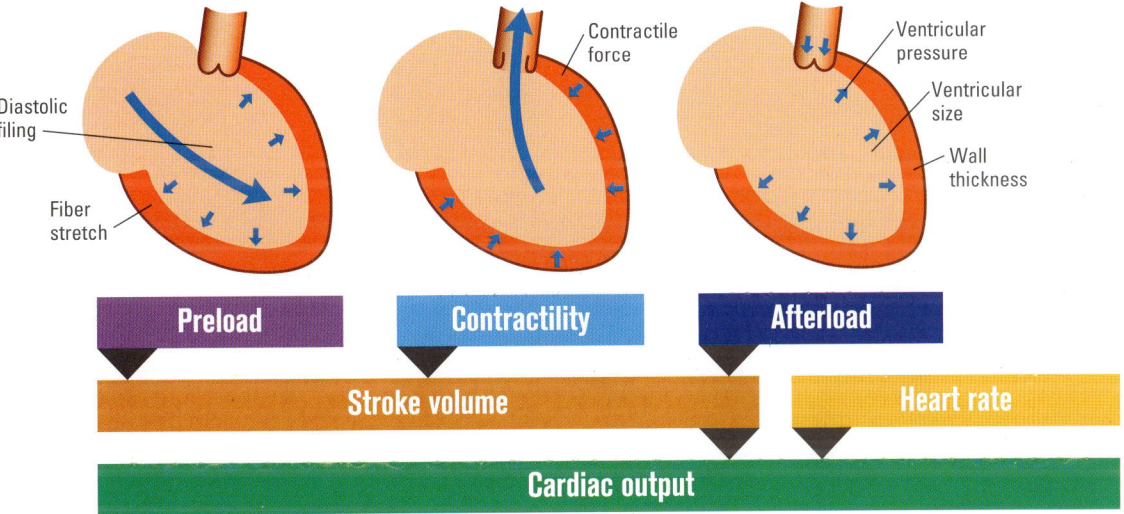

Understanding preload, contractility, and afterload

If you think of the heart as a balloon, it will help you understand preload, contractility, and afterload. (See the images that follow.)

Preload (blowing up the balloon)

Preload is the stretching of muscle fibers in the ventricle. This stretching results from blood volume in the ventricles at end diastole. According to Starling law, the more the heart muscles stretch during diastole, the more forcefully they contract during systole. Think of preload as the balloon stretching as air is blown into it. The more the air, the greater the stretch.

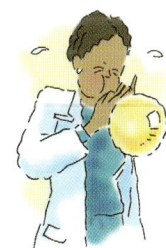

Contractility (the balloon's stretch)

Contractility refers to the inherent ability of the myocardium to contract normally. Contractility is influenced by preload. The greater the stretch, the more forceful the contraction—or, the more air in the balloon, the greater the stretch, and the farther the balloon will fly when air is allowed to expel.

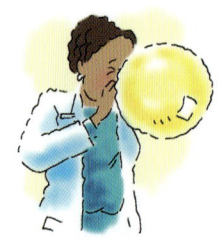

Afterload (the knot that ties the balloon)

Afterload refers to the pressure that the ventricular muscles must generate to overcome the higher pressure in the aorta to get the blood out of the heart. Resistance is the knot on the end of the balloon, which the balloon has to work against to get the air out.

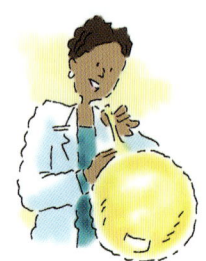

Effects of preload and afterload on the heart

Factor	Possible cause	Effects on heart
Increased preload	• Increased fluid volume • Vasoconstriction	• Increases stroke volume • Increases ventricular work • Increases myocardial O_2 requirements
Decreased preload	• Hypovolemia • Vasodilation	• Decreases stroke volume • Decreases ventricular work • Decreases myocardial O_2 requirements
Increased afterload	• Hypovolemia • Vasoconstriction	• Decreases stroke volume • Increases ventricular work • Increases myocardial O_2 requirements
Decreased afterload	• Vasodilation	• Increases stroke volume • Decreases ventricular work • Decreases myocardial O_2 requirements

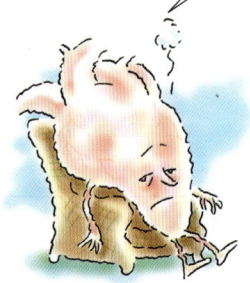

You can tell by looking at me what happens when my work increases.

Quick quiz

Color my world

Trace the path of blood flow through the heart. Color sections blue where deoxygenated blood flows and red where oxygenated blood flows.

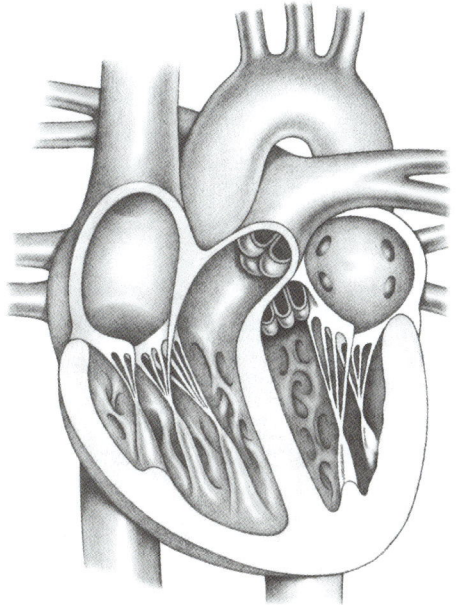

Matchmaker

Match each term to the appropriate definition.

1. Cardiac output _____   A. the pressure that the ventricular muscles must generate to overcome the higher pressure in the aorta.

2. Stroke volume _____   B. the stretching of muscle fibers in the ventricle.

3. Preload _____   C. the amount of blood the heart pumps in 1 minute.

4. Afterload _____   D. the amount of blood ejected with each heartbeat.

5. Contractility _____   E. the inherent ability of the myocardium to contract normally.

Answers: Color my world: See the illustration on page 9 for the correct path of flow and the correct colors; Matchmaker: 1. C, 2. D, 3. B, 4. A, 5. E

Selected references

Delgado, S. (2023). *AACN essentials of critical care nursing* (5th ed.). McGraw-Hill.

Diepenbrock, N. (2020). *Quick reference to critical care* (6th ed.). Lippincott Williams & Wilkins.

Hartjes, T. (Ed.). (2022). *Core curriculum for high acuity, progressive and critical care nursing* (8th ed). W.B. Saunders Co.

McLaughlin, M. A. (2025). *Cardiovascular care made incredibly easy* (5th ed). Wolters Kluwer.

Norris, T. L. (2025). *Porth's pathophysiology* (11th ed.). Wolters Kluwer.

Chapter 2

Understanding a pressure monitoring system

The purpose of a pressure monitoring system

Hemodynamic monitoring is used to:
- diagnose, manage, and treat cardiopulmonary insufficiency
- manage and treat shock
- assess pulmonary vascular function and blood flow
- assess cardiac function.

It's performed using a pressure monitoring system to measure cardiovascular pressures.

The components of a pressure monitoring system

A pressure monitoring system is made up of the components in the below figure (as described on the next page):

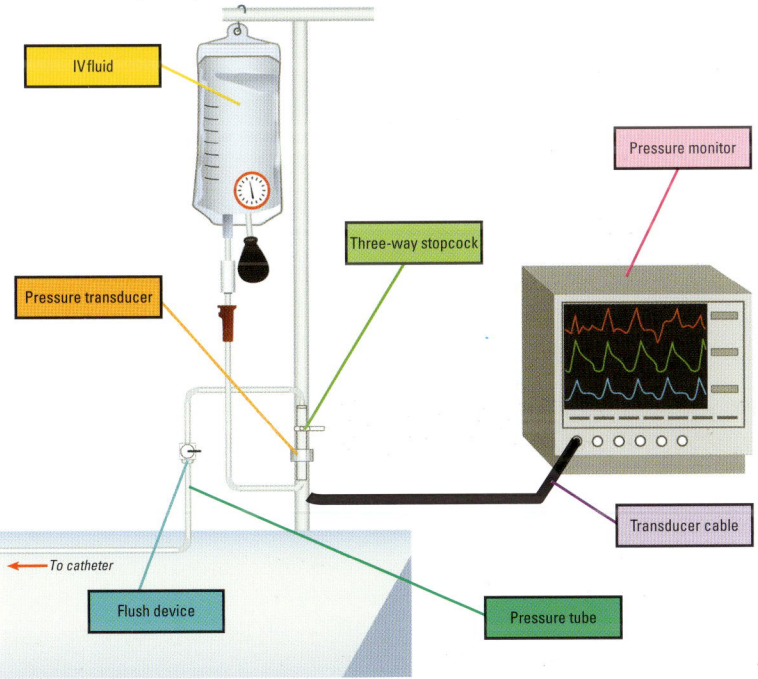

IV fluid

Pressure monitor

Three-way stopcock

Pressure transducer

Transducer cable

To catheter

Flush device

Pressure tube

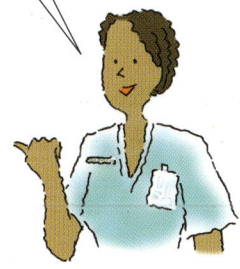

This system measures cardiac function and helps determine the effectiveness of therapy.

- **Pressure transducer**: The transducer senses pressure changes that are transmitted from the intravascular space or cardiac chamber to the fluid in the nonpliable pressure tubing through the catheter in the patient and from the nonpliable pressure tubing to the transducer. These pressure changes are transmitted to the monitor via electrical impulses sent through the transducer cable.
- **Flush device:** The flush device is used to manually flush the system.
- **IV fluid:** A continuous infusion of flush solution (usually normal saline or heparinized normal saline) is placed in a pressure bag that's inflated to 300 mm Hg, maintains a constant pressure through the transducer and flush device, and is kept at a low continuous flow of approximately 3 mL/hour to maintain patency, to prevent the back-flow of blood, and to allow for accurate pressure transmissions.
- **Pressure monitor:** The monitor converts the transducer's electrical signals into a pressure tracing (waveform) and digital value that are displayed on the screen.
- **Three-way stopcock:** The three-way stopcock is a device that controls the flow of IV solution through the system.
- **Pressure tube:** The pressure tubing serves as a connecting tube from the catheter in the patient to the flush device and transducer system. This tubing should be rigid and nonpliable to transmit the most accurate pressure measurements.
- **Transducer cable:** The transducer cable connects the pressure transducer to the monitor.

Multiple-pressure transducer systems

Multiple-pressure transducer systems can monitor two or more types of pressure, such as pulmonary artery pressure and central venous pressure. Two methods may be used to set up this type of system:

1. Add a second setup (with a separate bag of flush solution, pressure transducer, and cable) to the single-pressure system. Label the lines.
2. Use a Y-type tubing setup with two attached pressure transducers, requiring only one bag of flush solution but two pressure cables.

Leveling the transducer

Understanding leveling

To ensure accurate hemodynamic measurements, the patient and the transducer must be positioned on the same level before the system is zeroed. Leveling involves positioning the air-reference stopcock or the air-fluid interface of the transducer on the same level as the phlebostatic axis. Alternatively, the air-reference stopcock or the air-fluid interface may be leveled to the same position as the catheter tip.

How to level the transducer

Follow these steps to level the transducer:

1. **Determine the phlebostatic axis.** The phlebostatic axis (level of the patient's atria) is the zero-referencing point for the pressure monitoring system. The patient should be lying flat in bed, and the axis is established midway between the posterior chest and the sternum at the fourth intercostal space.

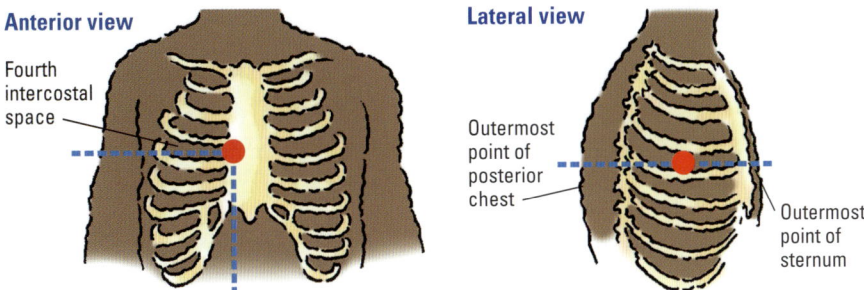

2. **Level the system.** Using a carpenter's level, place the air-reference stopcock or the air-fluid interface of the transducer on the same horizontal level as the phlebostatic axis.

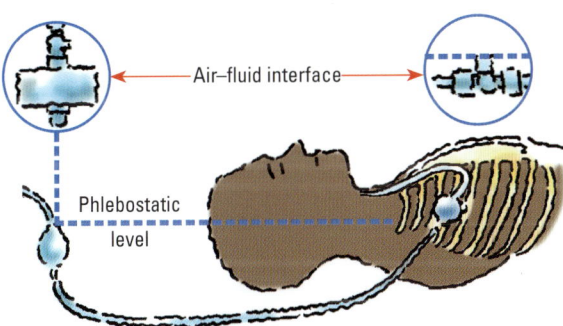

Nurses use a lot of tools—even a carpenter's level comes in handy for hemodynamic monitoring!

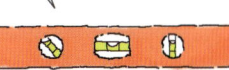

3. **Readjust as necessary.** If the head of the patient's bed is changed (raised or lowered), remember that the reference level will also change. Relevel and zero the system to allow for accurate measurements.

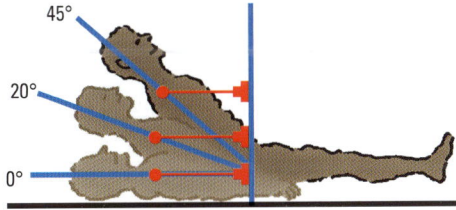

Effects of position changes on hemodynamic measurements

Catheter tip and transducer dome at the same vertical level

When the transducer is precisely aligned to midchest, there are no effects of hydrostatic pressure on the transducer diaphragm, and the displayed intravascular or intracardiac pressures are accurate.

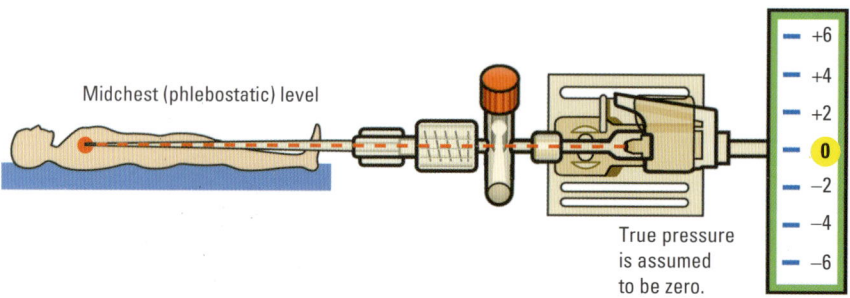

Midchest (phlebostatic) level

True pressure is assumed to be zero.

+6
+4
+2
0
−2
−4
−6

Air-fluid interface 3 inches below catheter tip

For every inch the transducer is below midchest level, the weight of the fluid on the transducer diaphragm will add 2 mm Hg to the true intravascular or intracardiac pressure.

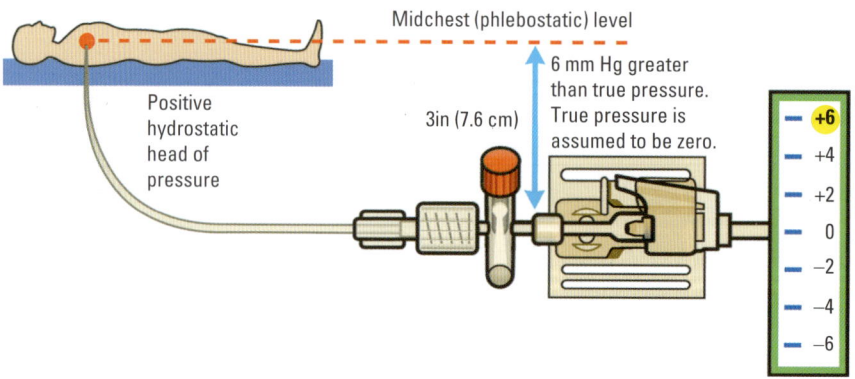

Midchest (phlebostatic) level

Positive hydrostatic head of pressure

3in (7.6 cm)

6 mm Hg greater than true pressure. True pressure is assumed to be zero.

+6
+4
+2
0
−2
−4
−6

Air-fluid interface 3 inches above catheter tip

For every inch the transducer is above midchest level, the displayed intravascular or intracardiac pressure will be about 2 mm Hg less than actual pressures.

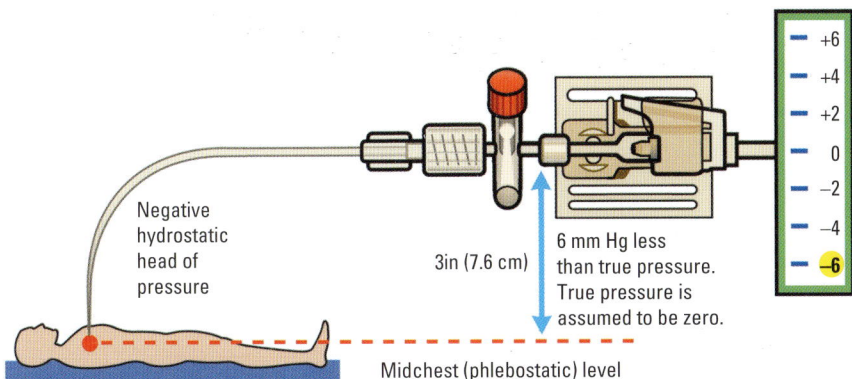

Negative
hydrostatic
head of
pressure

3in (7.6 cm)

6 mm Hg less
than true pressure.
True pressure is
assumed to be zero.

Midchest (phlebostatic) level

+6
+4
+2
0
−2
−4
−6

Zeroing the transducer

Understanding zeroing

After the pressure monitoring system is leveled, it's time to zero the transducer. Zeroing adjusts the transducer so that it reads zero pressure when it's open to the atmosphere. Zeroing is important because physiologic pressures, such as arterial blood pressure, are relative to the atmospheric pressure. By zeroing the transducer, effects from atmospheric pressure are eliminated, and the monitoring system begins pressure measurement at a neutral pressure point of 0 mm Hg. Establishing this neutral point ensures that pressure measurements reflect only the pressure values in the vessel or heart chamber being monitored.

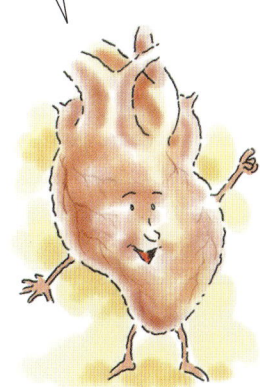

Zeroing the
transducer ensures
that pressure
measurements
reflect only the
pressure values in one
of my chambers.

How to zero the transducer

Follow these steps to zero the transducer:
1. Level the transducer.
2. Turn the stopcock next to the transducer off to the patient and open to air.
3. Remove the cap from the stopcock port and place it inside an opened sterile gauze package to prevent contamination.
4. Zero the transducer by activating the zero function key on the monitor.
5. When the monitor indicates the system is properly zeroed, replace the stopcock port cap and turn the stopcock so that it's closed to air and open to the patient. Now the monitoring can begin!

Square wave testing

The square wave test is a simple process performed to evaluate the dynamic response of the pressure monitoring system. If the waveform obtained when performing this test is optimal, you can be assured that the pressure monitoring system is providing accurate pressures and waveforms from the patient.

Performing and interpreting the square wave test

The square wave test is performed by activating the fast-flush device for 1 to 2 seconds and immediately evaluating the configuration on the monitor. The patient's pressure waveform displayed on the monitor will be replaced with a square wave.

Optimally damped system

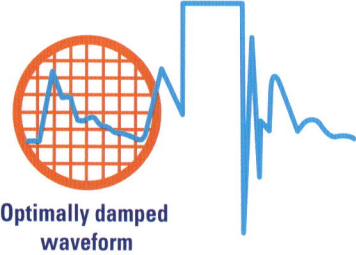

**Optimally damped
waveform**

Characteristics
- Straight vertical upstroke from the baseline
- Straight horizontal component
- Straight vertical downstroke back to baseline with one or two rapid oscillations (most important component).

Interventions
- None required.

Overdamped system

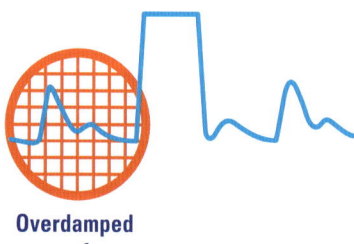

**Overdamped
waveform**

Characteristics

- Slurred upstroke and downstroke of the square wave
- No oscillations above or below the baseline.

Interventions

- Examine the system from the catheter to the transducer, checking for and eliminating blood clots, blood left in the catheter or tubing following sampling, or air bubbles at any point.
- Be sure to use nonpliable (stiff), pressurized tubing that's less than 4 in (1.2 m) long.
- Make sure that all components of the system are connected securely; unravel any kinks in the tubing.

Underdamped system

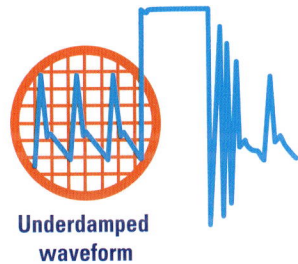

Underdamped waveform

Characteristics

- Numerous oscillations above and below baseline after activation of the fast-flush device.

Interventions

- Examine the tubing and remove all air bubbles from the fluid system.

Troubleshooting the pressure monitoring system

The table that follows provides helpful hints for troubleshooting the pressure monitoring system.

Problem	Possible causes	Nursing interventions
No waveform	• Power supply turned off • Monitor screen pressure range set too low • Loose connection in line • Transducer not connected to amplifier • Stopcock off to patient • Catheter occluded or out of blood vessel	• Check the power supply. • Raise the monitor screen pressure range if necessary. • Rebalance and recalibrate the equipment. • Tighten loose connections. • Position the stopcock correctly. • Use the fast-flush valve to flush the line, or try to aspirate blood from the catheter. If the line remains blocked, notify the provider and prepare to replace the line.

(continued)

Problem	Possible causes	Nursing interventions
Drifting waveforms	• Improper warm-up • Electrical cable kinked or compressed • Temperature change in room air or IV flush solution	• Allow the monitor and transducer to warm up for 10–15 minutes. • Place the monitor's cable where it can't be stepped on or compressed. • Routinely zero and calibrate the equipment 30 minutes after setting it up to allow IV fluid to warm to room temperature.
Line fails to flush	• Stopcocks positioned incorrectly • Inadequate pressure from pressure bag • Kink in pressure tubing • Blood clot in catheter	• Make sure stopcocks are positioned correctly. • Make sure the pressure bag gauge reads 300 mm Hg. • Check the pressure tubing for kinks. • Try to aspirate the clot with a syringe. If the line still won't flush, notify the provider and prepare to replace the line, if necessary. **Important:** Never use a syringe to flush a hemodynamic line.
Artifact (waveform interference)	• Patient movement • Electrical interference • Catheter fling (tip of pulmonary artery catheter moving rapidly in large blood vessel or heart chamber)	• Wait until the patient is quiet before taking a reading. • Make sure electrical equipment is connected and grounded correctly. • Notify the doctor, who may try to reposition the provider.
False-high readings	• Transducer balancing port positioned below patient's right atrium • Flush solution flow rate is too fast. • Air in system • Catheter fling (tip of pulmonary artery catheter moving rapidly in large blood vessel or heart chamber)	• Position the balancing port level with the patient's right atrium. • Check the flush solution flow rate. Maintain it at 3–4 mL/hour. • Remove air from the lines and the transducer. • Notify the doctor, who may try to reposition the catheter.
False-low readings	• Transducer balancing port positioned above right atrium • Transducer imbalance • Loose connection	• Position the balancing port level with the patient's right atrium. • Make sure the transducer's flow system isn't kinked or occluded, and rebalance and recalibrate the equipment. • Tighten loose connections.
Damped waveform	• Air bubbles • Blood clot in catheter • Blood flashback in line • Incorrect transducer position • Arterial catheter out of blood vessel or pressed against vessel wall	• Secure all connections. • Remove air from the lines and the transducer. Check for and replace cracked equipment. • Try to aspirate the clot with a syringe. If the line still won't flush, notify the doctor and prepare to replace the line, if necessary. Important: Never use a syringe to flush a hemodynamic line. • Make sure stopcock positions are correct; tighten loose connections and replace cracked equipment; flush the line with the fast-flush valve; and replace the transducer dome if blood backs up into it. • Make sure the transducer is kept at the level of the right atrium at all times. Improper levels give false-high or false-low pressure readings. • Reposition the catheter if it's against the vessel wall. Try to aspirate blood to confirm proper placement in the vessel. If you can't aspirate blood, notify the doctor and prepare to replace the line. **Note:** Bloody drainage at the insertion site may indicate catheter displacement. Notify the doctor immediately.

Quick quiz

Able to label?

Label the pieces of equipment in a pressure monitoring system indicated on this illustration.

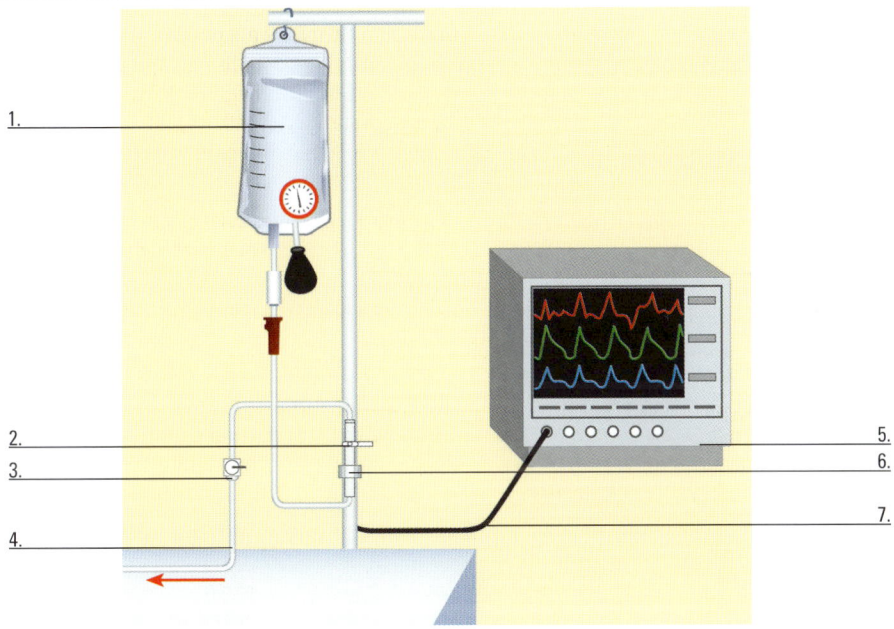

1. _____
2. _____
3. _____
4. _____
5. _____
6. _____
7. _____

Matchmaker

Match the following pressure monitoring problems with their causes:

1. No waveform _____

2. Drifting waveform _____

3. Lines fail to flush _____

4. Artifact _____

5. False-high readings _____

6. False-low readings _____

7. Dampened waveform _____

A. air bubbles

B. transducer imbalance

C. flush solution flow rate too fast

D. stopcocks positioned incorrectly

E. electrical interference

F. loose connection in line

G. kinked electrical cable

Answers: Able to Label?: Refer to the figure on page 19;
Matchmaker: 1. F, 2. G, 3. D, 4. E, 5. C, 6. B, 7. A

Selected references

Delgado, S. (2023). *AACN essentials of critical care nursing* (5th ed.). McGraw-Hill.

Diepenbrock, N. (2020). *Quick reference to critical care* (6th ed.). Lippincott Williams & Wilkins.

Hartjes, T. (Ed.). (2022). *AACN core curriculum for critical care nursing* (8th ed.). Elsevier.

Johnson, K. (Ed.). (2023). *AACN procedure manual for progressive and critical care* (8th ed.). Elsevier.

McLaughlin, M. A. (2025). *Cardiovascular care made incredibly easy* (5th ed.). Wolters Kluwer.

Chapter 3

Vascular access

Arterial line insertion

An arterial line provides access for invasive arterial pressure monitoring (e.g., continuous blood pressure monitoring) and can be used to obtain blood samples when frequent blood draws are indicated, including arterial blood gases.

A closer look at arterial insertion sites

Typically, a standard 18G to 20G over-the-needle catheter is inserted into a peripheral artery, usually the radial, brachial, or femoral artery. The radial artery is the preferred site.

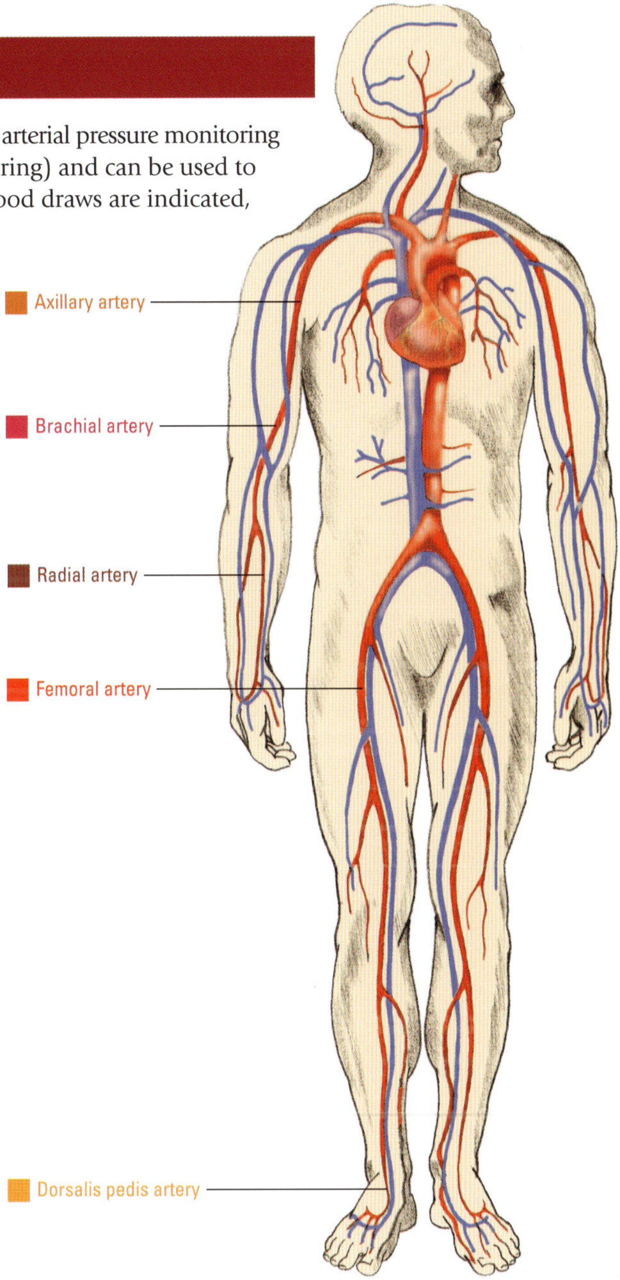

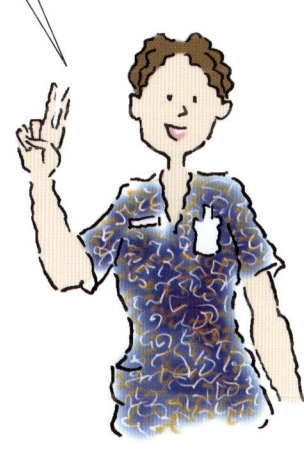

Arterial line insertion occurs most frequently in the radial or femoral artery.

■ Axillary artery

■ Brachial artery

■ Radial artery

■ Femoral artery

■ Dorsalis pedis artery

Choosing an arterial catheter site

When your patient needs arterial pressure monitoring, an arterial catheter will probably be inserted in the radial artery. If these sites are unsuitable, the catheter may be inserted in the femoral, brachial, axillary, or dorsalis pedis artery. Regardless of the site chosen, it should have an artery large enough to accommodate the arterial catheter without impeding distal blood flow. It should also be free of infection or traumatic injury proximal to the insertion site. The insertion can also be facilitated using ultrasound-guided vascular access.

Advantages and disadvantages of each site are described in the following table.

Insertion site	Advantages	Disadvantages
Radial artery	• Easy to locate • Good collateral circulation to the hand provided by the ulnar artery • Easy to observe and maintain • Anatomically stable (The radius acts as a natural splint.) • Comfortable for the patient	• Relatively small lumen, possibly making catheter insertion difficult and painful • High risk of thrombus formation with prolonged use due to the small vessel size and small-gauge catheter required to cannulate it • Risk of nerve injury due to hematoma formation or trauma during catheter insertion • Risk of false high-pressure readings because of the site's distance from the heart
Brachial artery	• Larger than the radial artery and easily located • Easy to observe and maintain • Good collateral circulation provided by blood vessels at the elbow joint • Control or prevention of bleeding usually possible by direct pressure	• Risk of median nerve damage during catheter insertion • Difficult to immobilize (The patient's elbow must be splinted, which may result in joint stiffness.) • Risk of thrombosis if the artery is small (in children and small women) or if the patient has low cardiac output.
Femoral artery	• Possibly the easiest artery to locate and puncture during an emergency (when peripheral pulses are nonpalpable) because of its large lumen • Anatomically stable (The femur acts as a natural splint.)	• Difficult catheter insertion in the presence of atherosclerotic plaque (In addition, the plaques may embolize if disturbed.) • Possible damage to the nearby femoral vein and major nerves during catheter insertion • Possible tissue damage if the artery occludes because of inadequate collateral circulation • Difficulty securing catheter • Difficulty controlling or preventing bleeding • High risk of infection with prolonged use because of close proximity to perineal area

Insertion site	Advantages	Disadvantages
Axillary artery	• Fewer complications with prolonged use because of large size • Reduced risk of distal arterial insufficiency because of adequate collateral blood flow • Useful in patients with severe peripheral vascular disease	• Difficult catheter insertion and uncomfortable for the patient • Risk of hematoma formation increases the possibility of neurovascular complications. • Risk of cerebral air or clot embolism during flushing of the system or blood sampling
Dorsalis pedis artery	• May be used when other sites cannot be used because of burns or other injuries.	• High risk of thrombosis because of the small vessel size and small-gauge catheter required for insertion • Uncomfortable for the patient and difficult to immobilize (The patient will not be able to stand or walk until the catheter is discontinued.)

Allen test

Before accessing the radial artery for peripheral arterial line insertion, the patient's ulnar and radial circulation must be checked for collateral circulation. Why? If the radial artery is blocked by a blood clot (a common complication of arterial lines), the ulnar artery alone must supply blood to the hand. A simple, reliable test of circulation can be done by performing the Allen test, which demonstrates how well both arteries supply blood to the hand.

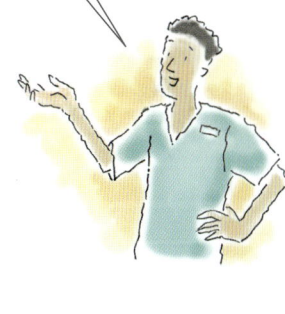

Remember: Use the Allen test to ensure that, if the radial artery is blocked, the ulnar artery will be able to supply blood to the hand.

Performing the Allen test

Follow these steps to perform the Allen test:
1. Rest the patient's arm on a flat surface, such as having the patient rest their arm at their side on the mattress or on the bedside stand. Support the patient's wrist with a rolled towel. Have them clench their fist. Then, using your index and middle fingers, palpate and then press both the radial and ulnar arteries. Hold this position for a few seconds.

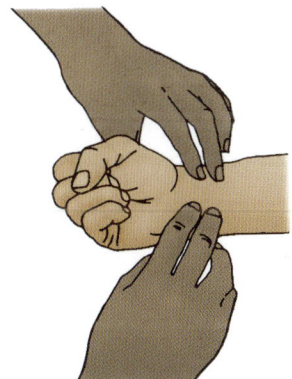

2. Without removing your fingers from the patient's arteries, ask them to unclench their fist and hold their hand in a relaxed position. The palm will be blanched because pressure from your fingers has impaired the normal blood flow.

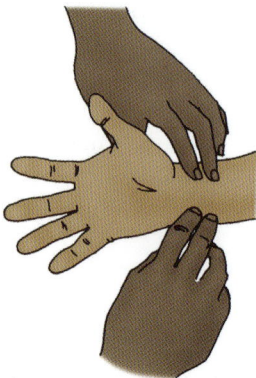

3. Release pressure on the patient's ulnar artery but keep pressure on the radial artery, as shown below. Observe the palm for a brisk return of color or "flushing," which should occur within 7 seconds (showing a patent ulnar artery and adequate blood flow to the hand). If color returns in 7 to 15 seconds, blood flow is impaired; if color returns after 15 seconds, consider the flow inadequate.

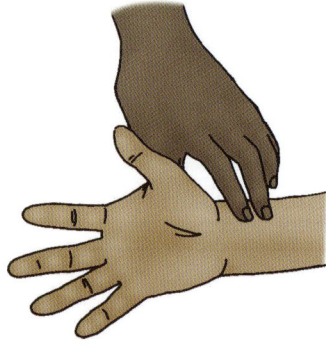

   If blood flow is impaired or inadequate, the radial artery in this hand should not be used. At this point, proceed with the Allen test on the other hand. If neither hand colors or flushes, consider another site, such as the brachial artery, for catheter insertion.

Caring for arterial catheters

There are three steps to basic care for arterial catheters:

1. **Dressing:** After insertion of the arterial catheter, dress the insertion site and change it according to facility policy. Sterile dressing changes are recommended. Transparent dressings are typically

used over the insertion site to enable complete visualization of the site. This breathable film allows oxygen in and moisture vapors out, while also providing barrier protection.

2. **Immobilizing:** The body part where the catheter is placed will then need to be immobilized. The joint or limb should be placed in a neutral position to prevent joint flexion or extension, which may result in kinking or dislodgment of the catheter. If the radial artery has been used, take care not to hyperextend the wrist, which could result in nerve or neuromuscular injury. Assess the limb with the arterial cannulation for any associated pressure points when immobilizing the extremity. Regularly assess the functioning of the arterial line to prevent kinking.

3. **Assessing:** The arterial catheter site must be assessed every hour. Include the following in your assessment:
    ◆ Inspect the arterial catheter insertion site for redness, drainage, bruising, or blanching. (The benefit of using a transparent dressing becomes apparent at this step.) Palpate the area for firmness or swelling.
    ◆ Assess circulation of the extremity in which the arterial catheter has been placed by evaluating skin color, temperature, capillary refill, distal pulses (if applicable), and motor and sensory function.

A closer look at an arterial line

This photograph shows an arterial line taped in place in the radial artery. (Flush is shown in Chapter 4.)

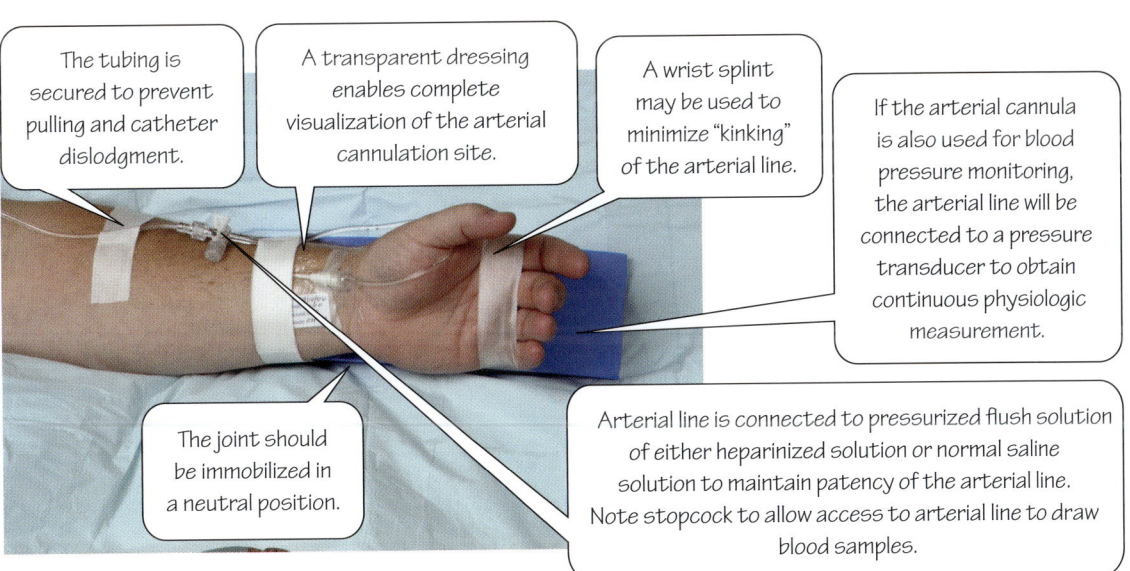

The tubing is secured to prevent pulling and catheter dislodgment.

A transparent dressing enables complete visualization of the arterial cannulation site.

A wrist splint may be used to minimize "kinking" of the arterial line.

If the arterial cannula is also used for blood pressure monitoring, the arterial line will be connected to a pressure transducer to obtain continuous physiologic measurement.

The joint should be immobilized in a neutral position.

Arterial line is connected to pressurized flush solution of either heparinized solution or normal saline solution to maintain patency of the arterial line. Note stopcock to allow access to arterial line to draw blood samples.

Central venous and pulmonary artery catheter insertion

Central venous and pulmonary artery catheter insertion sites

The most common sites for percutaneous insertion of a central venous (CV) or pulmonary artery (PA) catheter include the internal jugular, subclavian, and femoral veins. The right internal jugular vein is considered the safest insertion site. Although the subclavian vein is easily accessed, its use carries certain risks. The most significant risk is pneumothorax, resulting from puncturing the lung at a level above the clavicle during catheter insertion. In addition, using the subclavian vein may cause the catheter or the introducer to bend or kink during insertion. Although the femoral vein is easily accessible, use of this site carries an increased risk of infection because of the proximity to the groin.

Other access sites may include the antecubital vein.

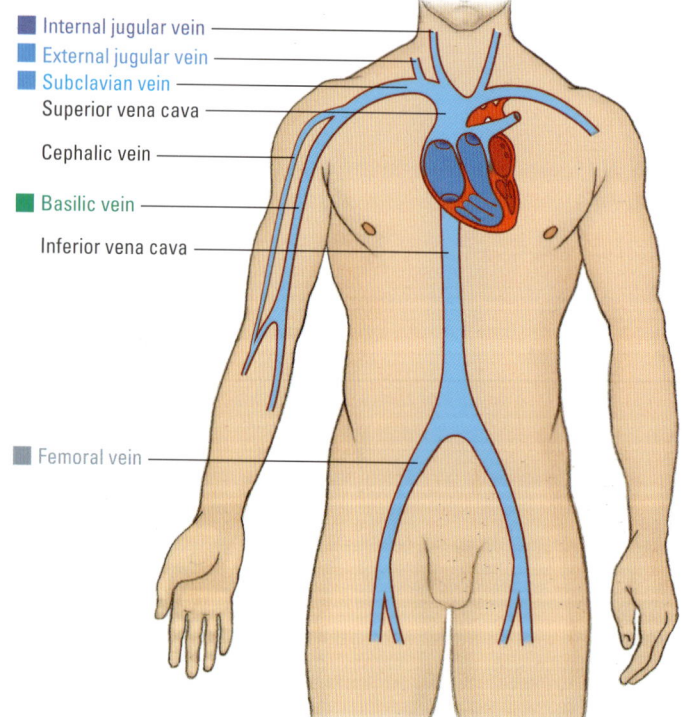

- Internal jugular vein
- External jugular vein
- Subclavian vein
- Superior vena cava
- Cephalic vein
- Basilic vein
- Inferior vena cava
- Femoral vein

Central venous and pulmonary artery catheterization

CV and PA catheterization can help you assess a patient's cardiovascular and pulmonary status, obtain blood samples, and infuse solutions. Inserted in a surgical, sterile procedure in the jugular, subclavian, femoral, or basilic vein, the catheter is flow directed, allowing venous circulation to carry it through to a position in or near the right atrium (for CV catheters) or through the right atrium and ventricle to the PA (for PA catheters).

Placement can be guided by ultrasound using transthoracic echocardiography or radiographic imaging using fluoroscopy. In addition, the provider inserting the PA catheter will be guided by waveforms as the catheter transverses through the right atrium, right ventricle, and into the PA.

Choosing a central venous or pulmonary artery catheter insertion site

The following table highlights the advantages and disadvantages of the most common sites used for CV or PA catheter insertion. Catheter-related infection is the most common risk at every insertion site, occurring in up to 5% of cases.

Insertion site	Advantages	Disadvantages

Internal jugular vein	• Provides a short, direct route to the superior vena cava or right atrium
	• Carries a low risk of catheter displacement
	• Has a lower incidence of pneumothorax or perforation of an artery than with a subclavian vein
	• Has a lower risk of thrombotic complications because rapid infusion rates may be used
		• Several complications, including:
		  • air embolism
		  • common carotid artery perforation
		  • perforation of the trachea or endotracheal (ET) tube cuff
		  • pneumothorax (more common in the left internal jugular vein)
		  • injury to the thoracic duct (applicable only to left internal jugular vein)

Externa jugular vein (peripheral access)	• Is easily accessible because of its superficial location
	• Carries a low risk of pneumothorax or puncture of the carotid artery
		• Difficult passage to the central veins
		• Increased risk of thrombosis because infusion rates must be slower
		• Difficulty maintaining a sterile dressing, especially with the presence of a tracheostomy
		• Several possible complications, including:
		  • carotid artery perforation
		  • pneumothorax
		  • displacement into axillary vein

Subclavian vein	• Is easily accessible
	• Enables easy maintenance of a sterile, intact dressing
	• Allows the patient to move their neck and arm freely
	• Carries minimal risk of catheter displacement after it is secured
	• Carries a reduced risk of thrombosis because rapid infusion rates are allowable
		• Several possible complications, including:
		  • air embolism
		  • subclavian artery perforation
		  • life-threatening blood loss (because pressure cannot be applied to an anterior subclavian tear)
		  • pneumothorax
		  • phrenic or brachial nerve injury
		  • ET tube cuff perforation

Insertion site	Advantages	Disadvantages

Femoral vein	• Is easily accessible
	• Enables greater ease of insertion in patients with tortuous subclavian and jugular veins (such as in older adult patients)
	• Carries no risk of pneumothorax and a minimal risk of air embolism
		• Possibly difficult to identify in patients with obesity
		  • Increased risk of infection because of proximity to the groin
		  • Difficulty maintaining a sterile, intact dressing
		  • Increased risk of catheter displacement because the site is difficult to immobilize
		  • Several possible complications, including:
		    • inadvertent cannulation of local smaller veins
		    • thrombosis

Basilic vein (peripheral access)	• Carries no risk of pneumothorax or major hemorrhage
	• Enables greater control in bleeding from the site
		• Difficult to identify in patients who are obese or edematous
		• Possible difficulty advancing the catheter to the central veins from this distal site
		• Increased risk of catheter displacement
		• Several possible complications, including:
		  • thrombosis
		  • venous spasm

Insertion of the catheter

Before catheter insertion, assess the patient's vital signs, obtain consent and explain the procedure, and set up the appropriate tubing.

CV and PA catheters share the same approaches to insertion—a surgical cutdown technique or a percutaneous technique using sterile technique.

A surgical cutdown involves identifying the vein to be used for insertion, administering a local anesthetic, and making a small incision directly above the vessel. The catheter is then inserted by direct needle puncture of the vessel, or by creating a tiny incision in the vessel, through which the catheter is inserted and then sutured in place. Surgical cutdown is typically performed for central catheters inserted through the basilic vein or when percutaneous access is not possible.

Introducer kit

The more commonly used percutaneous technique involves the use of an introducer to access the vessel. A locator needle is first inserted in the vein, and a guide wire is threaded through the needle. The needle is removed, and an introducer catheter is inserted over the wire. Then, the wire is removed, leaving the introducer in place in the blood

> No matter which technique you use to insert a CV or PA catheter, it should be performed under strict sterile conditions.

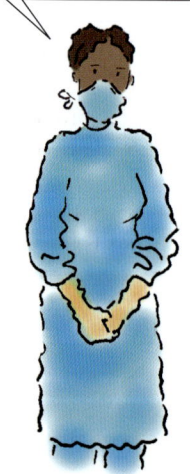

vessel. The CV or PA catheter is then inserted through the introducer sheath. Prepackaged introducer kits, such as the one shown below, are available to facilitate gathering and preparation of equipment.

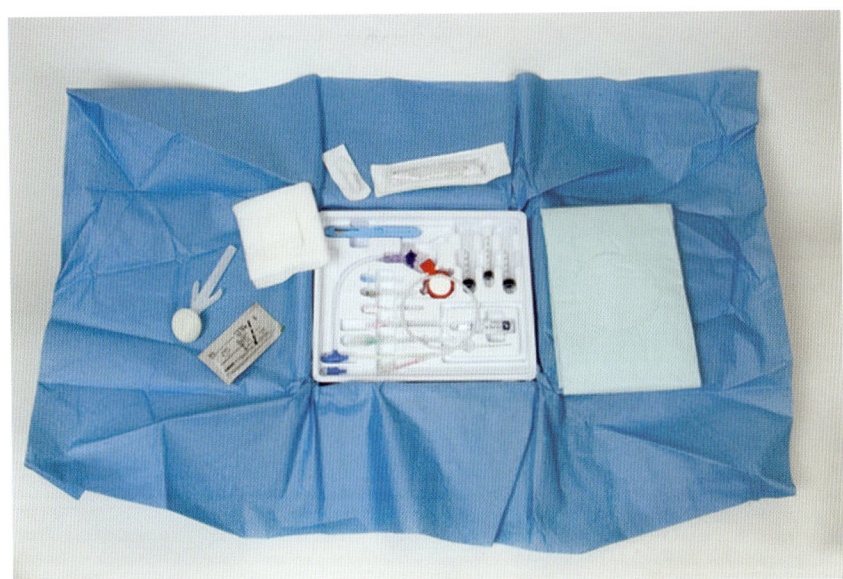

Patient positioning

Proper patient positioning during CV or PA catheter insertion is essential to enable optimal access to the site and prevent contamination. These guidelines will help you position your patient depending on the insertion site you are using:

- Place the patient in the Trendelenburg position to dilate the veins and reduce the risk of air embolism. (This position is not necessary if you are using the femoral vein site.)
- For subclavian insertion, place a rolled blanket or towel lengthwise between the shoulders to increase venous distention.
- For jugular insertion, place a rolled blanket or towel under the opposite shoulder to extend the neck, making anatomic landmarks more visible.
- Have the patient wear a mask or turn the patient's head away from the insertion site to prevent possible contamination from airborne pathogens and to make the site more accessible.

Positioning for subclavian vein access

For subclavian vein access, in addition to placing a rolled blanket or towel lengthwise between the patient's shoulders, the patient should be positioned with head turned away from the access site with the chin pointed upward, as shown here. In addition, have the patient wear a mask to reduce risk of insertion site infection.

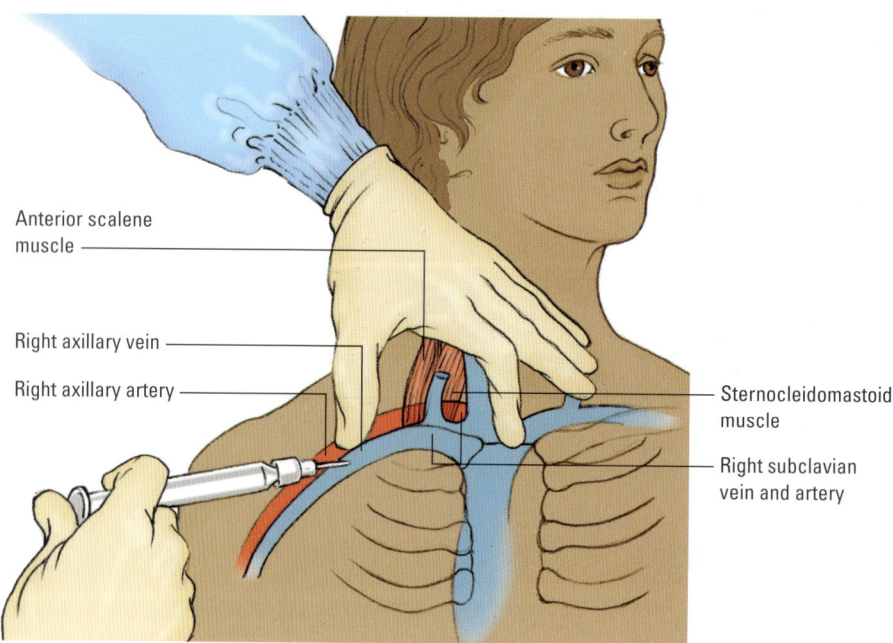

Potential complications during insertion or after placement

Potential complications of a PA or central venous pressure (CVP) catheter during insertion may include pneumothorax, air embolism, arterial puncture, or bleeding. In addition, cardiac dysrhythmias may occur during PA catheter insertion. After-placement complications of CVP and PA catheters can include thrombosis and infection.

A closer look at catheter insertion

The following photographs show a PA catheter being inserted through an introducer during a percutaneous insertion procedure.

1. After the introducer is in place, the PA catheter may be inserted.

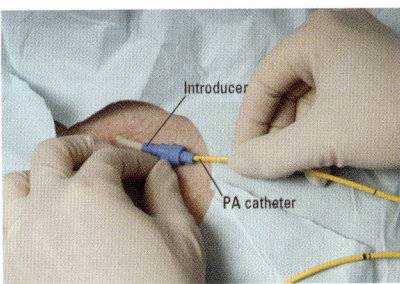

2. Because the introducer completely occupies the puncture sites at the skin and blood vessel, there is minimal bleeding from the site.

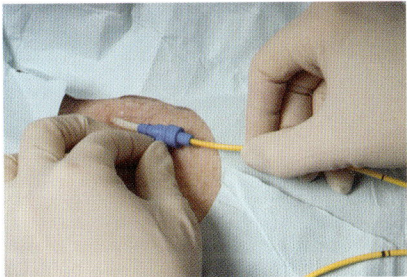

3. The PA catheter is inserted 5″ to 6″ to reach the superior vena cava from the internal jugular or right subclavian insertion sites. A longer length is required from the femoral site.

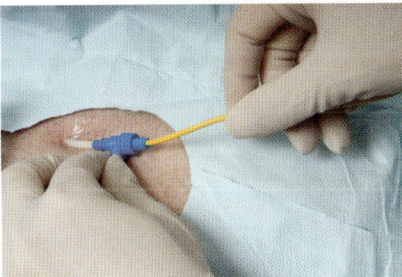

Changing a central venous dressing

According to the Centers for Disease Control and Prevention (CDC), expect to change your patient's CV dressing every 48 hours if it is a gauze dressing and at least every 5 to 15 days if it is transparent or if the integrity of the dressing is compromised. Sterile dressing changes are indicated whenever the dressing becomes soiled, moist, or loose. The following illustrations show the key steps you will perform.

1. Put on a mask and clean gloves and remove the old dressing (as shown below) by pulling it toward the exit site of a long-term catheter or toward the insertion site of a short-term catheter. This technique helps you avoid pulling out the line. If a chlorhexidine disk is in place, remove it. Remove and discard your gloves.

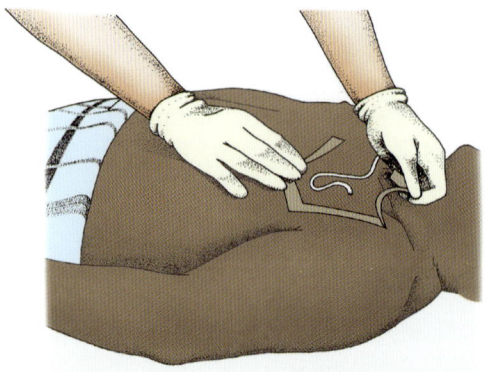

2. Put on sterile gloves and clean the skin around the catheter with an antimicrobial skin cleanser (usually chlorhexidine), using a vigorous side-to-side motion (as shown below).

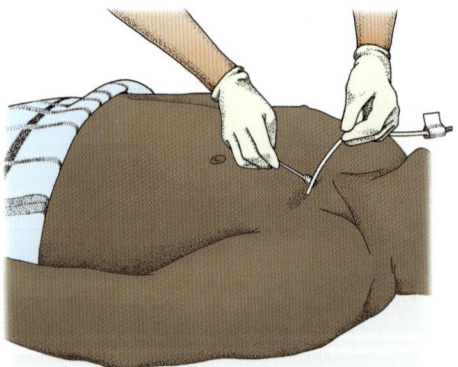

3. Allow the skin to dry completely. Apply a new chlorhexidine disk if indicated.
4. After the solution has dried, cover the site with a dressing, such as a transparent semipermeable dressing. Write the time and date on the dressing. Document the dressing change including the appearance of the catheter insertion site.

Indications for central venous pressure or pulmonary artery catheter

Both types of catheters can be very useful to evaluate volume status in patients who are acutely ill. The catheters can also be useful in determining whether the patient has fluid-volume status changes and left ventricular heart dysfunction. The PA catheter can specifically provide continuous monitoring of the PA pressure and can be used to obtain cardiac output. The pressure monitoring provided by the CVP or PA catheter can be useful in guiding the use of fluid therapy and/or vasoactive medication (e.g., dopamine) titration.

Quick quiz

Able to label?

In the illustration, label the arterial insertion sites.

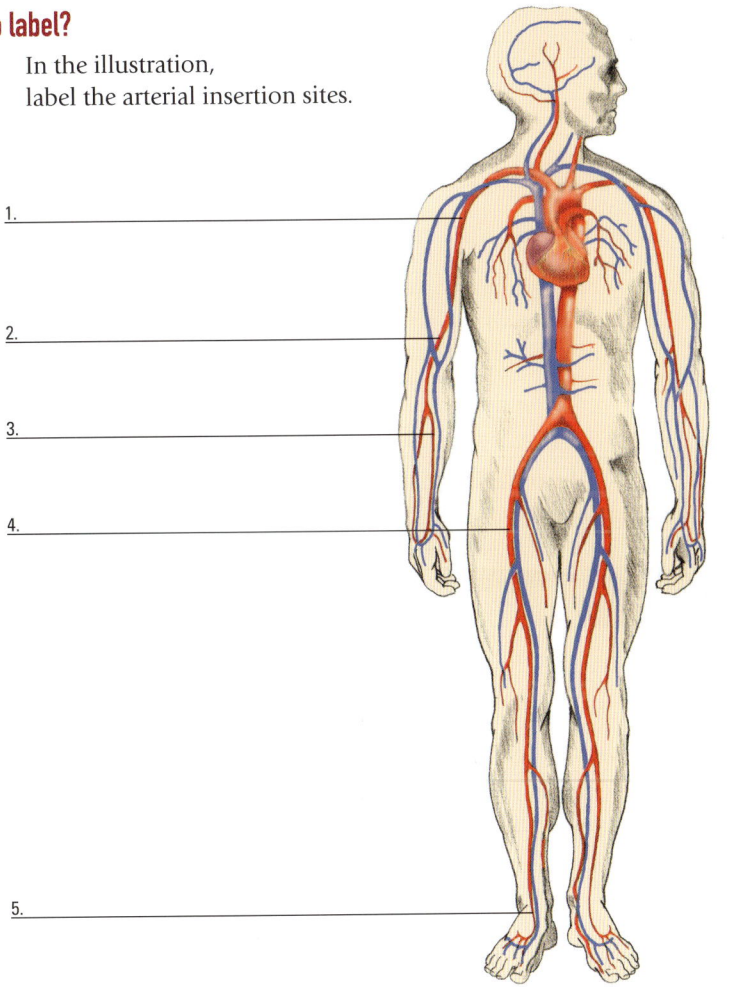

1. _____

2. _____

3. _____

4. _____

5. _____

True or false

1.   An arterial line can measure CVP.

2.   Flush solutions used to maintain patency of arterial lines ALWAYS REQUIRE heparin.

Multiple choice

1.   Which of the following is the most common insertion site for arterial cannulation?
  A.   ulnar artery
  B.   brachial artery
  C.   radial artery
  D.   internal carotid artery

2.   When a PA catheter is used to obtain a pulmonary artery wedge pressure (PAWP), an indirect pressure reading is obtained for which of the following?
  A.   left atrial pressure
  B.   pulmonary arterial pressure
  C.   superior vena cava pressure
  D.   coronary artery pressure

3.   Which of the following parameters can be obtained from the PA catheter?
  A.   blood pressure
  B.   stroke volume
  C.   oxygen saturation
  D.   pulmonary artery mean pressure

Answers: Able to label? 1. Axillary artery, 2. Brachial artery, 3. Radial artery, 4. Femoral artery, 5. Dorsal pedis artery; True or false: 1. False, 2. False; Multiple choice: 1. C, 2. A, 3. D

Selected references

Delgado, S. A. (2023). *AACN essentials of critical care nursing* (5th ed.). McGraw-Hill.

Diepenbrock, N. (2020). *Quick reference to critical care* (6th ed.). Wolters Kluwer.

Hartjes, T. (Ed.). (2022). *Core curriculum for critical care nursing* (8th ed.). Elsevier.

Johnson, K. (Ed.). (2023). *AACN procedure manual for high acuity, progressive, and critical care* (8th ed.). Elsevier.

McLaughlin, M. A. (2025). *Cardiovascular care made incredibly easy* (5th ed.). Wolters Kluwer.

Morton, P. G., & Fontaine, D. K. (2023). *Critical care nursing: A holistic approach* (12th ed.). Wolters Kluwer.

Perpetua, E., & Keegan, P. (2021). *Cardiac nursing* (7th ed.). Lippincott Williams & Wilkins.

Ramírez, M., Mazwi, M. L., Bronicki, R. A., Checchia, P. A., & Ong, J. S. M. (2023). Beyond conventional hemodynamic monitoring-monitoring to improve our understanding of disease process and interventions. *Critical Care Clinics*, 39(2), 243–254. https://doi.org/10.1016/j.ccc.2022.09.002

Chapter 4

Arterial pressure monitoring

Arterial pressure monitoring basics

Arterial pressure monitoring measures arterial pressure directly, using an indwelling arterial catheter connected to an external pressure transducer and fluid-filled tubing. The tubing is attached to a pressure bag of saline or heparin flush solution, and the transducer is attached to a monitor. The pressure transducer converts the pressure into an electrical signal that is interpreted and displayed on a monitor screen as a continuous waveform. The pressure may also be shown as a digital readout.

The radial artery is the preferred site of catheter insertion because this artery is readily accessible. However, brachial, axillary, femoral, or pedal artery may also be used.

Hand hygiene and the use of personal protective equipment (mask, goggles, gloves) are essential in preventing infection.

A closer look at an arterial pressure monitoring system

The figure on these pages shows an arterial pressure monitoring system:

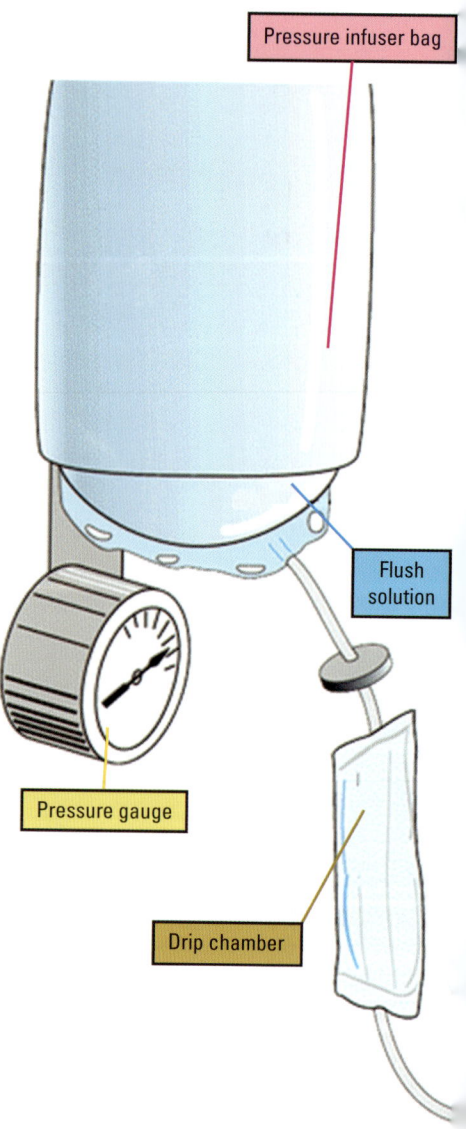

Pressure infuser bag

Flush solution

Pressure gauge

Drip chamber

Uses of arterial pressure monitoring

Direct arterial pressure monitoring permits continuous measurement of systolic, diastolic, and mean pressures and allows arterial blood sampling. Because direct measurement reflects systemic vascular resistance as well as blood flow, it is generally more accurate than are indirect methods based on blood flow (such as palpation and auscultation for Korotkoff sounds). Moreover, direct arterial pressure monitoring aids in determining mean arterial pressure (MAP), an important indicator of tissue perfusion.

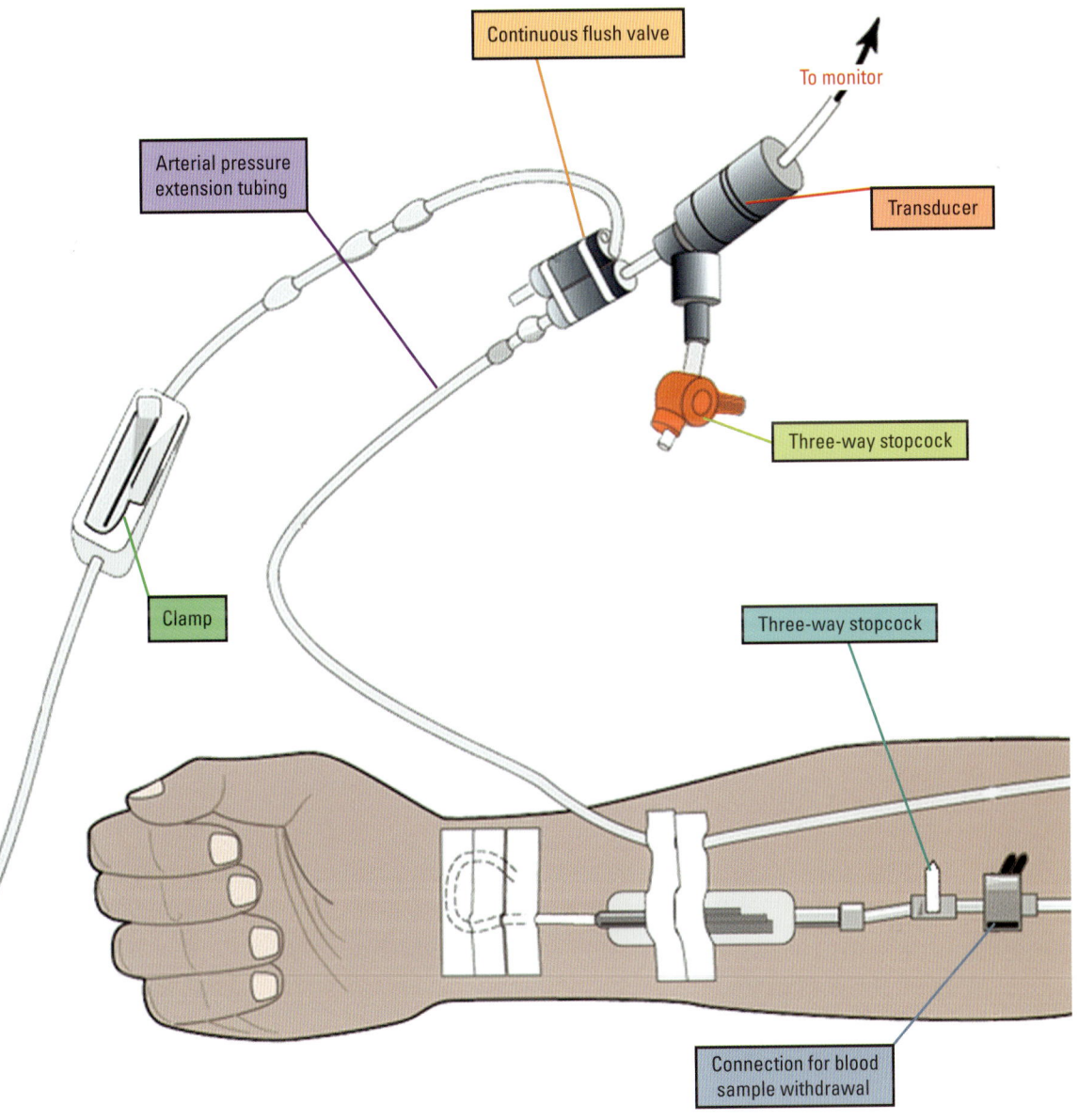

Continuous flush valve

To monitor

Arterial pressure
extension tubing

Transducer

Three-way stopcock

Clamp

Three-way stopcock

Connection for blood
sample withdrawal

Indications and contraindications

Indications for arterial blood pressure monitoring include the following:
- when highly accurate or frequent blood pressure measurements are required
- for patients receiving doses of vasoactive drugs requiring titration
- for patients requiring frequent blood sampling.

Relative contraindications for arterial blood pressure monitoring include:
- peripheral vascular disease
- hemorrhagic disorders
- use of anticoagulants or thrombolytic agents.

Insertion site contraindications for arterial blood pressure monitoring include:
- areas of active infection or with synthetic graft materials
- sites of prior vascular surgery.

 **On the level**

Normal arterial pressure parameters

In general, arterial systolic pressure reflects the peak pressure generated by the left ventricle. It also indicates compliance of the large arteries, or the peripheral resistance.

Arterial diastolic pressure reflects the runoff velocity and elasticity of the arterial system, particularly of the arterioles.

MAP is the average pressure in the arterial system during systole and diastole. It reflects the driving, or perfusion, pressure and is determined by arterial blood volume and blood vessel elasticity and resistance. To compute MAP, use this formula:

$$MAP = \frac{Systolic\ pressure + 2\ (Diastolic\ pressure)}{3}$$

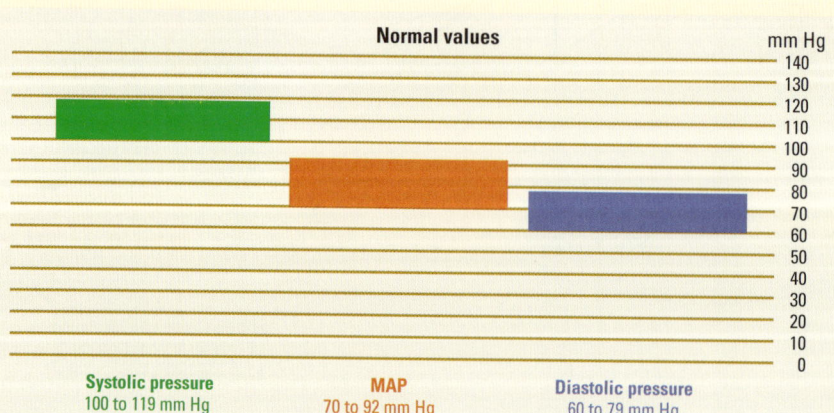

Normal values

		mm Hg

Systolic pressure
100 to 119 mm Hg

MAP
70 to 92 mm Hg

Diastolic pressure
60 to 79 mm Hg

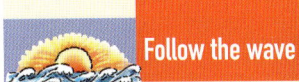

Follow the wave

Understanding an arterial waveform

Normal arterial blood pressure produces a characteristic waveform representing ventricular systole and diastole. The waveform has five distinct components:

- anacrotic limb
- systolic peak
- dicrotic limb
- dicrotic notch
- end diastole.

The anacrotic limb marks the waveform's initial upstroke, which results as blood is rapidly ejected from the ventricle through the open aortic valve into the aorta. The rapid ejection causes a sharp rise in arterial pressure, which appears as the waveform's highest point. This point is called the *systolic peak*.

As blood continues into the peripheral vessels, arterial pressure falls and the waveform begins a downward trend. This part is called the *dicrotic limb*. Arterial pressure usually continues to fall until pressure in the ventricle is less than the pressure in the aortic root. When this unequal pressure occurs, the aortic valve closes. This event appears as a small notch on the waveform's downside, known as the *dicrotic notch*.

When the aortic valve closes, diastole begins, progressing until the aortic root pressure gradually descends to its lowest point. On the waveform, this is known as *end diastole*.

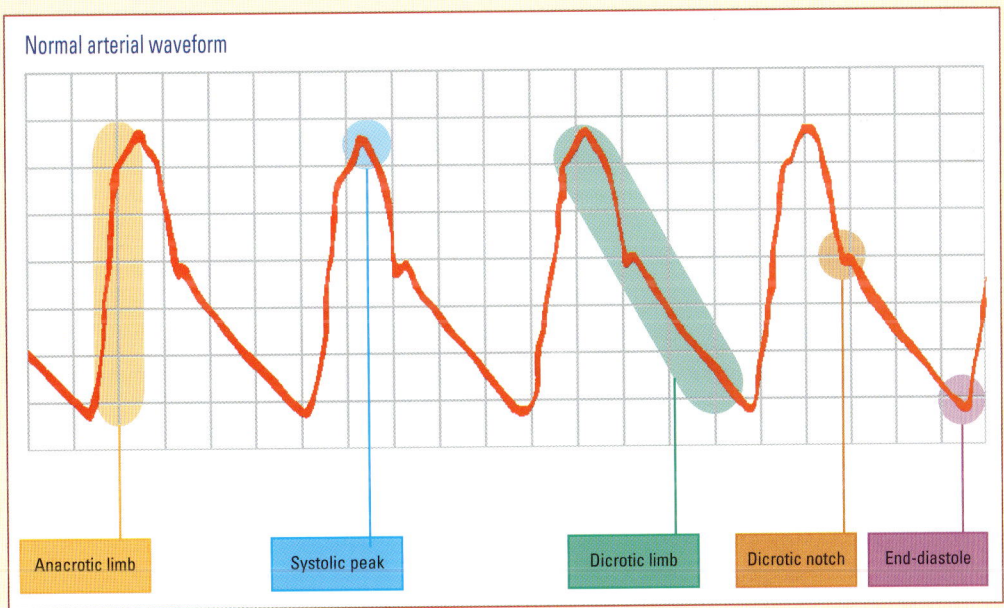

Normal arterial waveform

| Anacrotic limb | Systolic peak | Dicrotic limb | Dicrotic notch | End-diastole |

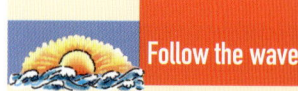

Follow the wave

Recognizing abnormal arterial waveforms

Understanding a normal arterial waveform is relatively straightforward. Unfortunately, an abnormal waveform is not so easy to decipher. Abnormal patterns and markings, however, may provide important diagnostic clues to the patient's cardiovascular status, or they may simply signal trouble in the monitor. Use this chart to help you recognize and resolve waveform abnormalities.

Waveform	Abnormality
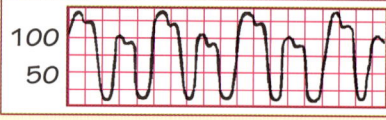	Alternating high and low waves in a regular pattern
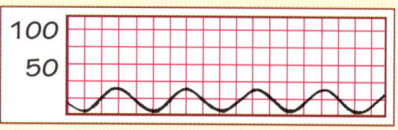	Flattened waveform
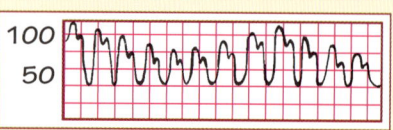	Slightly rounded waveform with consistent variations in systolic height
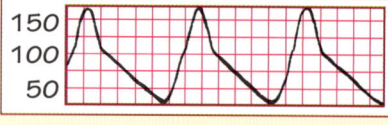	Slow upstroke
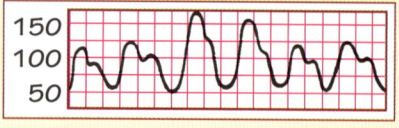	Diminished amplitude on inspiration
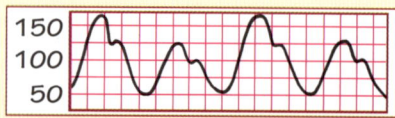	Alteration in beat-to-beat amplitude (in otherwise normal rhythm)

Possible causes	Nursing interventions
• Ventricular bigeminy	• Check the patient's electrocardiogram (ECG) to confirm ventricular bigeminy. The tracing should reflect premature ventricular contractions every second beat.
• Overdamped waveform or hypotensive patient	• Check the patient's blood pressure with a sphygmomanometer. If you obtain a higher reading, suspect overdamping. Correct the problem by trying to aspirate the arterial line. If you succeed, flush the line. If the reading is very low or absent, suspect hypotension.
• Patient on ventilator with positive end-expiratory pressure	• Check the patient's systolic blood pressure regularly. The difference between the highest and the lowest systolic pressure reading should be <10 mm Hg. If the difference exceeds that amount, suspect pulsus paradoxus, possibly from cardiac tamponade.
• Aortic stenosis	• Check the patient's heart sounds for signs of aortic stenosis. Also notify the provider, who will document suspected aortic stenosis in their notes.
• Pulsus paradoxus, possibly from cardiac tamponade, constrictive pericarditis, or lung disease	• Note systolic pressure during inspiration and expiration. If inspiratory pressure is at least 10 mm Hg less than expiratory pressure, call the doctor. • If you are also monitoring pulmonary artery pressure, observe for a diastolic plateau. This abnormality occurs when the mean central venous pressure (right atrial pressure), mean pulmonary artery pressure, and mean pulmonary artery wedge pressure (pulmonary artery obstructive pressure) are within 5 mm Hg of one another.
• Pulsus alternans, which may indicate left ventricular failure	• Observe the patient's ECG, noting any deviation in the waveform. • Notify the doctor if this is a new and sudden abnormality.

Zeroing the system

Because it is fluid filled, an arterial pressure monitoring system must be zeroed. Remember that zeroing balances the transducer to atmospheric pressure, so that it reads 0 mm Hg when open to air. The procedure for zeroing the monitoring system is described in detail in Chapter 2. The following photographs highlight some of the key steps in the procedure because it is performed on a peripheral arterial line.

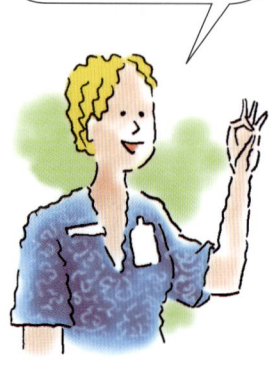

When it comes to accurate arterial pressure monitoring, zero is the magic number!

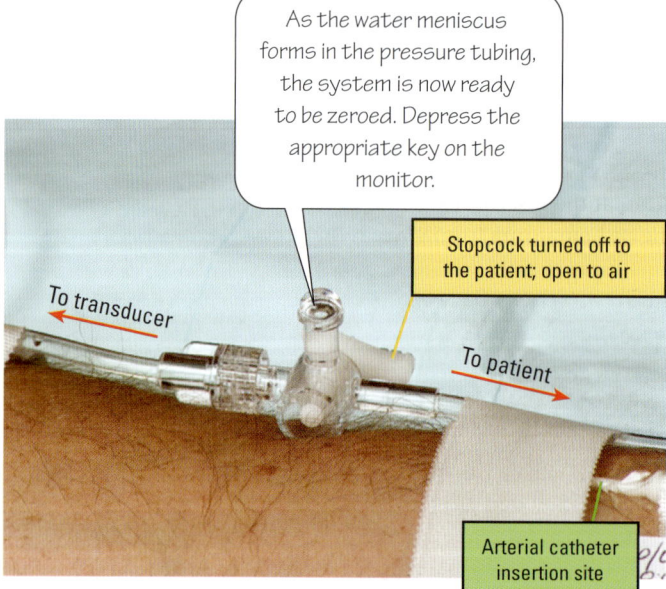

Stopcock turned off to the patient, open to air

Arterial catheter insertion site

As the water meniscus forms in the pressure tubing, the system is now ready to be zeroed. Depress the appropriate key on the monitor.

To transducer

Stopcock turned off to the patient; open to air

To patient

Arterial catheter insertion site

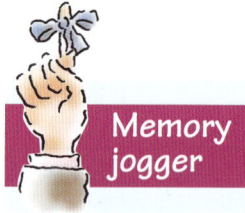

Memory jogger

When it comes to zeroing the system, remember that **zero equals none**. The transducer should read 0 mm Hg so that there is zero difference between the transducer pressure and the atmospheric pressure.

Managing issues related to arterial pressure monitoring

How to handle a displaced arterial line

Your patient is in danger of hypovolemic shock from blood loss if their arterial line is pulled out or otherwise displaced. Follow these steps to handle a displaced arterial line.

After the bleeding stops

- Withdraw blood for a complete blood count and arterial blood gas analysis, as ordered.
- Assist the doctor as they insert another catheter. Make sure that the patient's arm is immobilized and that the tubing and catheter are secure.
- Estimate the amount of blood loss from your observations of the blood and from the changes in the patient's blood pressure and heart rate.
- Apply a sterile pressure dressing.
- Reassess the patient's level of consciousness (LOC) and orientation and offer reassurance.

What to do first

- Check the patient's intravenous (IV) line and, if ordered, increase the flow rate temporarily to compensate for blood loss.
- Immediately apply direct pressure at the insertion site and have someone summon the doctor. Because arterial blood flows under high intravascular pressure, be certain to maintain firm, direct pressure for a minimum of 5 minutes to encourage clot formation at the insertion site.

Ongoing care

- Frequently assess the patient's vital signs, LOC, skin color and temperature, and circulation at the insertion site and beyond.
- Watch for further bleeding or hematoma formation at the insertion site.
- When the patient's condition stabilizes, reduce the IV flow rate to the previous keep-vein-open level.

Minimizing complications of arterial pressure monitoring

For most critically ill patients, the advantages of arterial lines outweigh the disadvantages. However, because any invasive hemodynamic monitoring procedure poses some risk, you will need to watch your patient for complications that may result from an arterial line.

Complications and signs and symptoms	Possible causes	Nursing interventions	Prevention
Thrombosis • Loss or weakening of pulse below arterial line insertion site • Loss of warmth, sensation, color, and mobility in limb below insertion site • Damped or straight waveform on monitor display or printout	• Arterial damage during or after insertion • Sluggish flow rate of flush solution • Failure to heparinize flush solution adequately • Failure to flush catheter routinely and after withdrawing blood samples • Irrigation of clotted catheter with a syringe	• Notify the doctor. They may remove the line. • Document the complication and record your interventions.	• Check the patient's pulse rate immediately after catheter insertion, then once hourly. • Reduce injury to the artery by splinting the limb holding the line and by taping the catheter securely. • Check the flush solution's flow rate hourly; maintain the rate at 3–4 mL/hour. • Check the pressure infuser bag to make sure that pressure is maintained at 300 mm Hg. • Heparinize the flush solution according to facility policy. • Flush the catheter once hourly and after withdrawing blood samples. • Never irrigate an arterial catheter. You may flush a blood clot into the bloodstream.
Blood loss • Bloody dressing; blood flowing from disconnected line	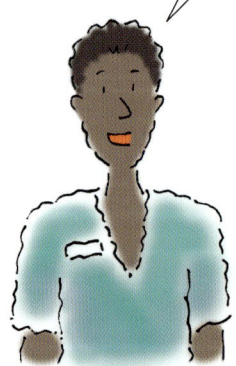 *A dislodged catheter or disconnected line could cause blood loss.*	• Stop the bleeding. • Check the patient's vital signs. • Notify the doctor if blood loss is great or if the patient's vital signs change. • If the line is disconnected, avoid reconnecting it. Instead, immediately replace contaminated equipment. • If the catheter is pulled out of the artery, remove it and apply direct pressure to the site; then notify the doctor. • When the bleeding stops, check the patient's pulse and the insertion site frequently for signs of thrombosis or hematoma. • Document the complication and record your interventions.	• Check the line connections and insertion site frequently. • Tape the catheter securely and splint the patient's limb. • Make sure that the monitor alarms are enabled.

Complications and signs and symptoms	Possible causes	Nursing interventions	Prevention
Air embolism or thromboembolism • Drop in blood pressure • Rise in central venous pressure • Weak, rapid pulse • Cyanosis • Loss of consciousness • Damped waveform	• Air in tubing • Loose connections	• Place the patient on their left side and in Trendelenburg position. If air has entered the heart chambers, this position may keep the air on the heart's right side. The pulmonary artery can then absorb the small air bubbles. • Check the arterial line for leaks. • Notify the doctor immediately, and check the patient's vital signs. • Administer oxygen if ordered. • Document the complication and record your interventions.	• Expel all air from the line before connecting it to the patient. • Make sure that all connections are secure; then check connections routinely. • Change the flush solution bag before it empties. • Prevent thromboembolism by keeping the arterial line patent with heparin flush solution.
Systemic infection • Sudden rise in temperature and pulse rate • Chills and shaking • Blood pressure changes	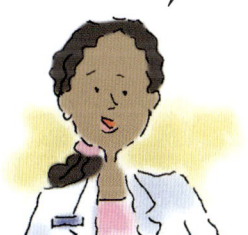 Causes may include poor aseptic technique, use of contaminated equipment, or irrigation of a clotted catheter.	• Look for other sources of infection first. Obtain urine, sputum, and blood specimens for cultures and other analyses, as ordered. • Notify the doctor. They may discontinue the line and send the equipment to the laboratory for study. • Document the complication and record your interventions.	• Review care procedures and ensure sterile technique. • Take care not to contaminate the arterial line insertion site when bathing the patient. • If any part of the line disconnects accidentally, do not rejoin it. Instead, replace the parts with sterile equipment. • Change system components as recommended (intravenous flush solution and pressure tubing every 96 hours, transparent dressing every 7 days, and nontransparent dressing every 24–48 hours).

Complications and signs and symptoms	Possible causes	Nursing interventions	Prevention
Arterial spasm • Intermittent loss or weakening of pulse below insertion site • Irregular waveform on monitor screen or printout	• Trauma to vessel during catheter insertion • Artery irritated by catheter after insertion	• Notify the doctor. • Prepare lidocaine (Xylocaine), which the doctor may inject directly into the arterial catheter to relieve the spasm. Caution: Make sure that a combination product containing lidocaine and epinephrine (Xylocaine with epinephrine) is not used; the epinephrine in this product could cause further arterial constriction. • Document the complication and record your interventions.	• Tape the catheter securely to prevent it from moving in the artery. • Splint the patient's limb to stabilize the catheter.
Hematoma • Swelling at insertion site and generalized swelling of limb holding arterial line • Bleeding at site	• Blood leakage around catheter (resulting from weakened or damaged artery) • Failure to maintain pressure at site after removing catheter	• Stop the bleeding. • If the hematoma appears while the catheter is in place, notify the doctor. • If the hematoma appears within 30 minutes of removing the catheter, apply ice to the site. • Otherwise, apply warm, moist compresses to help speed the hematoma's absorption. • Document the complication and record your interventions.	• Tape the catheter securely and splint the insertion area to prevent damage to the artery. • After the catheter is removed, apply firm, manual pressure over the site for a minimum of 5 minutes or until bleeding stops.
Inaccurate pressure readings **False-high values** • Transducer positioned too low • Small air bubbles in arterial line **False-low values** • Transducer positioned too high • Large air bubble in arterial line		• Relevel and rezero the transducer system. • Remove air bubbles. • Document the complication and record your interventions.	• Make sure to zero and calibrate the transducer system precisely. • Properly level the transducer at the level of the patient's right atrium (the phlebostatic axis). • Keep air from entering the pressure tubing or system. • Check the arterial waveform configuration for abnormalities.

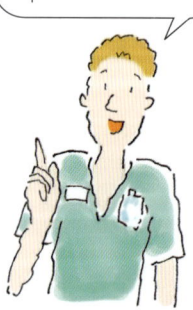

What's a sure sign of inaccurate pressure readings? Your patient's clinical appearance is inconsistent with pressure values.

Quick quiz

What do you know?

1. List six complications of arterial pressure monitoring.

_____   _____

_____   _____

_____   _____

2. Inaccurate pressure readings could be caused by an air bubble in what line?

_____

Matchmaker

Match the abnormal arterial waveforms in column 2 to their descriptions in column 1.

1. alternating high and low waves in a regular pattern _____

2. flattened waveform _____   A.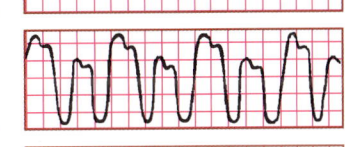

3. slightly rounded waveform with consistent variations in systolic height _____

   B.

4. slow upstroke _____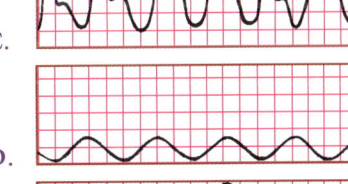

5. diminished amplitude on inspiration _____

6. alteration in beat-to-beat amplitude (in otherwise normal rhythm) _____   C.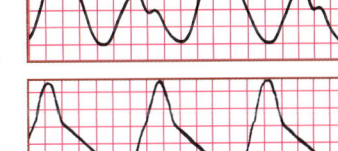

D.

E.

F.

Answers: What do you know?: 1. thrombosis, blood loss, embolism, hematoma, arterial spasm, systemic infection; 2. arterial.
Matchmaker: 1. B, 2. D, 3. A, 4. F, 5. C, 6. E

Selected references

Delgado, S. (2023). *AACN essentials of critical care nursing* (5th ed.). McGraw-Hill.

Diepenbrock, N. (2020). *Quick reference to critical care* (6th ed.). Lippincott Williams & Wilkins.

Hartjes, T. (Ed.). (2022). *AACN core curriculum for critical care nursing* (8th ed.). Elsevier.

Johnson, K. (2023). *AACN procedure manual for critical care* (8th ed.). Elsevier.

McLaughlin, M. A. (2025). *Cardiovascular care made incredibly easy* (5th ed.). Wolters Kluwer.

Morton, P. G., & Thurman, P. (2023). *Critical care nursing: A holistic approach* (11th ed.). Lippincott Williams & Wilkins.

O'Grady, N. P., Alexander, M., Burns, L. A., Dellinger, E. P., Garland, J., Heard, S. O., Lipsett, P. A., Masur, H., Mermel, L. A., Pearson, M. L., Raad, I. I., Randolph, A., Rupp, M. E., Saint, S., & Healthcare Infection Control Practices Advisory Committee. (2017). *Guidelines for the prevention of intravascular catheter-related infections (2011)*. Retrieved May 28, 2023, from https://www.cdc.gov/infectioncontrol/guidelines/BSI/index.html

Perpetua, E., & Keegan, P. (2021). *Cardiac nursing* (7th ed.). Lippincott Williams & Wilkins.

Chapter 5

Central venous pressure monitoring

Understanding central venous pressure monitoring

In central venous pressure (CVP) monitoring, the provider or licensed independent provider inserts a catheter through a vein and advances it until its tip lies in or near the right atrium. Because no major valves lie at the junction of the vena cava and right atrium, pressure at end diastole reflects directly back to the catheter. When connected to a transducer or manometer, the catheter measures CVP, a direct reflection of right atrial pressure and an indirect measure of preload of the right ventricle.

What it does

CVP monitoring helps assess cardiac function, evaluate venous return to the heart, and determine the volume status of the body. The central venous (CV) line also provides access to a large vessel for rapid, high-volume fluid administration and enables frequent blood withdrawal for laboratory samples. For patients who are critically ill, especially those in cariogenic shock, CVP is a marker for volume status.

Intermittent or continuous?

CVP monitoring can be done either intermittently or continuously. Typically, a single lumen CVP line is used for intermittent pressure readings using a disposable plastic water manometer. CVP is recorded in centimeters of water (cm H_2O) or millimeters of mercury (mm Hg) read from manometer markings. However, more commonly, a pressure transducer system is used to measure continuous CVP. It is vital to trend the CVP measurements rather than to obtain one single measurement, because the trend gives information about a patient's clinical status.

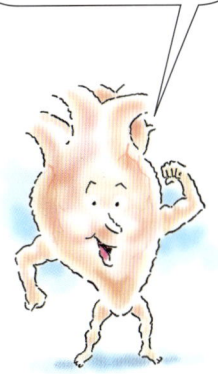

CVP helps indirectly gauge how well the heart—particularly the right side—is pumping.

A closer look at a central venous catheter

The below figure provides information about the parts of a CV catheter.

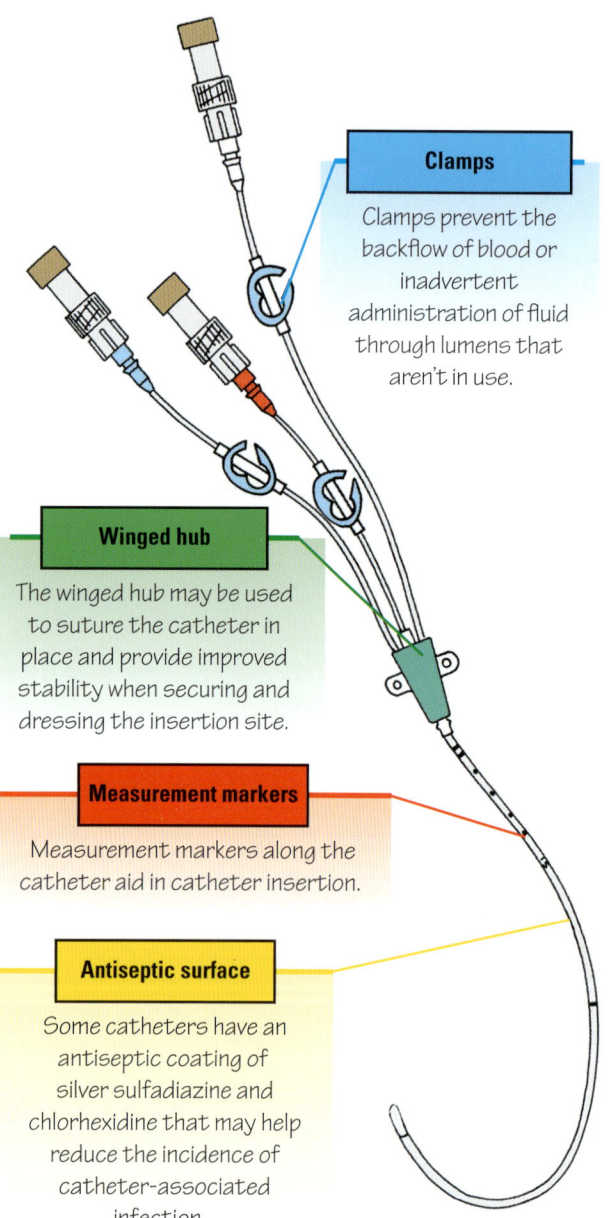

Clamps

Clamps prevent the backflow of blood or inadvertent administration of fluid through lumens that aren't in use.

Winged hub

The winged hub may be used to suture the catheter in place and provide improved stability when securing and dressing the insertion site.

Measurement markers

Measurement markers along the catheter aid in catheter insertion.

Antiseptic surface

Some catheters have an antiseptic coating of silver sulfadiazine and chlorhexidine that may help reduce the incidence of catheter-associated infection.

Obtaining CVP measurements

Follow these steps to obtain CVP measurements:

1. Make sure that the CV line or the proximal lumen of a pulmonary artery catheter is attached to the system. (If the patient has a CV line with multiple lumens, one lumen may be solely dedicated to continuous CVP monitoring and the other lumens may be used for fluid administration.)
2. Set up a pressure transducer system. Connect the nonpliable pressure tubing from the CVP catheter hub to the transducer. Then connect the flush solution container to a flush device.
3. To obtain values, position the patient flat. If they can't tolerate this position, elevate the bed to 30 degrees. Locate the level of the right atrium by identifying the phlebostatic axis. Zero the transducer, leveling the transducer air–fluid interface stopcock with the right atrium, as shown in the below photograph. Read the CVP value from the digital display on the monitor, and note the waveform. Make sure that the patient is still when the reading is taken to prevent artifact. Use this position (flat or 30 degrees) for all subsequent readings and when zeroing the transducer.

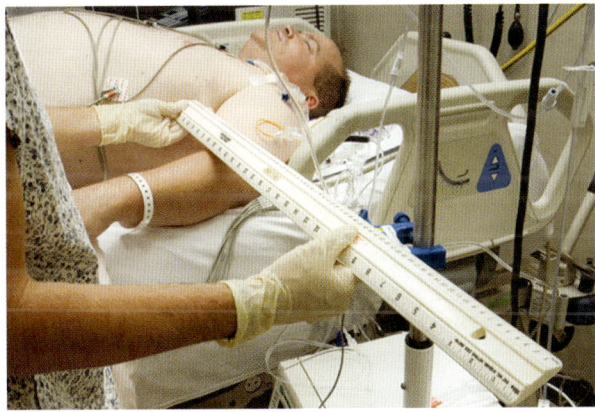

4. Intrathoracic pressure varies with respiration, which in turn impacts the CVP value. The ideal point in time at which to measure the CVP is at end expiration, when intrathoracic pressure is closest to atmospheric pressure.

Correlating CVP with cardiac function

Essentially, CVP measurements reflect events in the cardiac cycle and, thus, depict cardiac function. See the flow chart below for more information.

> During ventricular diastole, the atrioventricular (AV) valves open.

> As diastole ends, each open valve creates what amounts to a common heart chamber.

> The pressure created by blood volume in the ventricles then extends back into the atria so that pressure measured in the right atrium indirectly mirrors the volume status of the right ventricle (called *preload*).

> During systole, the AV valves close and the semilunar valves open.

> At this point, the pressure measured in the atria indicates atrial filling.

Central venous catheter pathways

The illustrations in this section show several common pathways for CV catheter insertion. Typically, a CV catheter is inserted in either the subclavian or internal jugular vein.

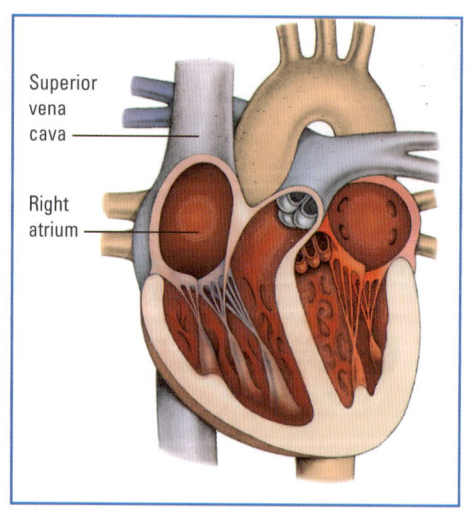

Superior vena cava

Right atrium

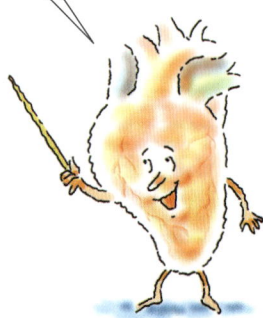

A CV catheter usually ends in the superior vena cava. However, it can also terminate in the right atrium.

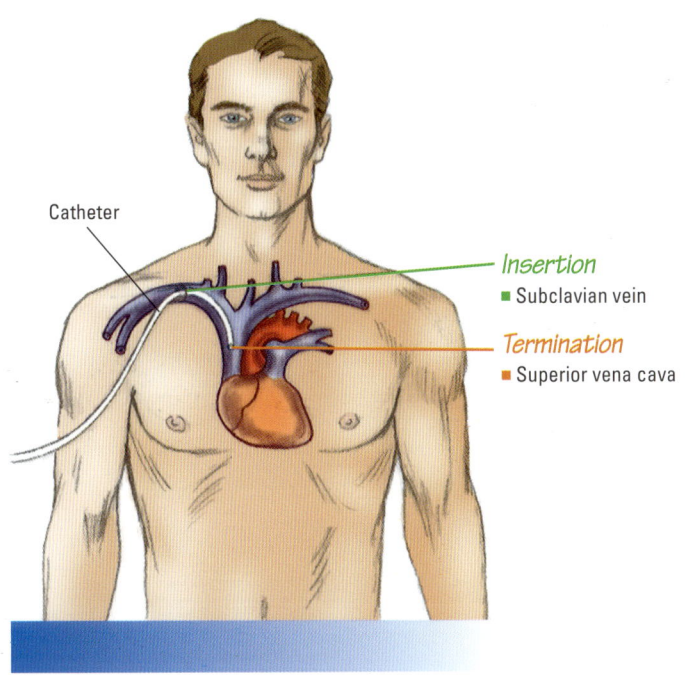

Catheter

Insertion
- Subclavian vein

Termination
- Superior vena cava

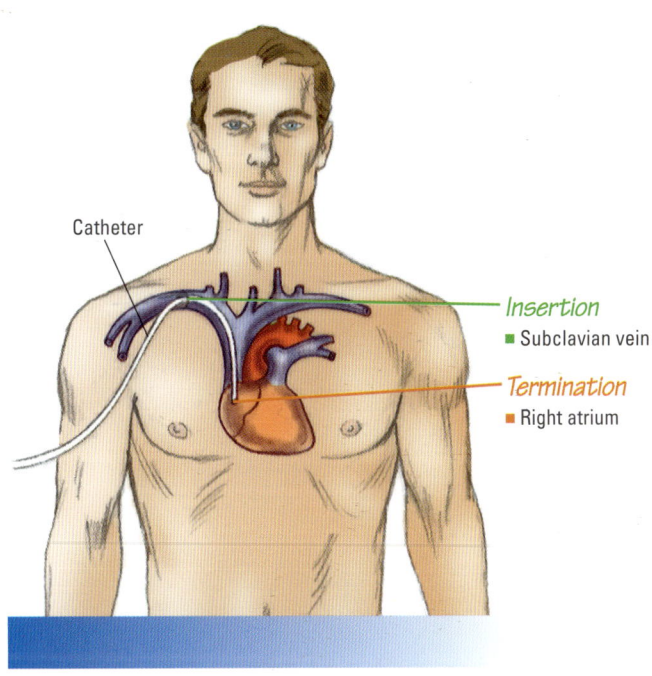

Catheter

Insertion
- Subclavian vein

Termination
- Right atrium

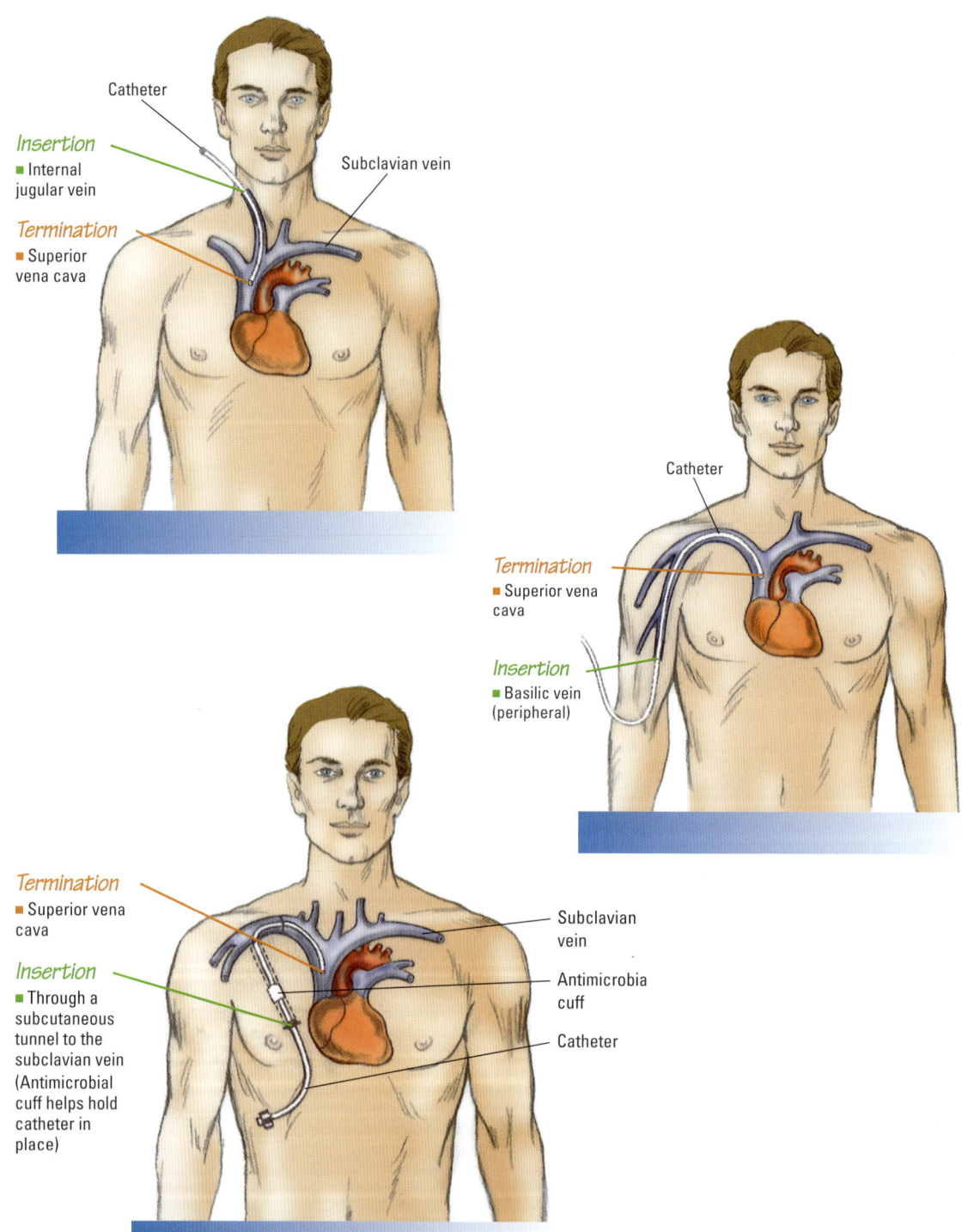

Catheter

Insertion
- Internal jugular vein

Subclavian vein

Termination
- Superior vena cava

Catheter

Termination
- Superior vena cava

Insertion
- Basilic vein (peripheral)

Termination
- Superior vena cava

Insertion
- Through a subcutaneous tunnel to the subclavian vein (Antimicrobial cuff helps hold catheter in place)

Subclavian vein

Antimicrobia cuff

Catheter

Follow the wave

Understanding the CVP waveform: Comparing electrical activity

When the CV catheter is attached to a pressure monitoring system, the bedside monitor can usually display digital pressure values, CVP waveforms, and electrocardiogram (ECG) tracings. Synchronizing the CVP waveform with the ECG helps you identify components of the tracing. Keep in mind that cardiac electrical activity precedes the mechanical activities of systole and diastole.

The **P** wave on the ECG reflects atrial depolarization, which is then followed by atrial contraction and increased atrial pressure. Corresponding to the PR interval on the ECG, the wave sequence on the CVP waveform represents atrial contraction.

The **x** descent on the CVP waveform represents atrial relaxation and declining pressure after systole, when the atrium expels blood into the ventricle. As the cardiac cycle progresses, the tricuspid valve closes, producing a small backward bulge known as the **c** wave.

The atrium filling with venous blood during diastole produces another rise in pressure and a **v** wave, which corresponds to the **T** wave of the ECG.

After atrial filling, the tricuspid valve opens. Most of the blood in the right atrium passively empties into the right ventricle, causing atrial pressure to fall. On the CVP waveform, this decline appears as the **y** descent.

The **a** and **v** waves are almost the same height, indicating that atrial systole and atrial diastole produce about the same amount of pressure. Consequently, right atrial pressures are recorded as mean values because they are almost the same.

Follow the wave

Normal CVP waveforms

The following figures show normal waveforms.

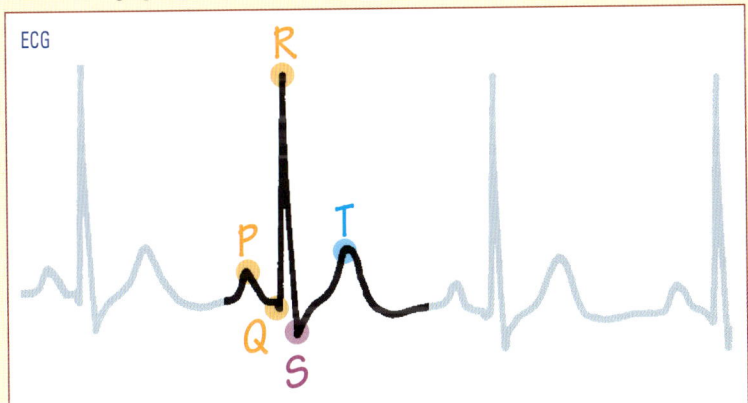

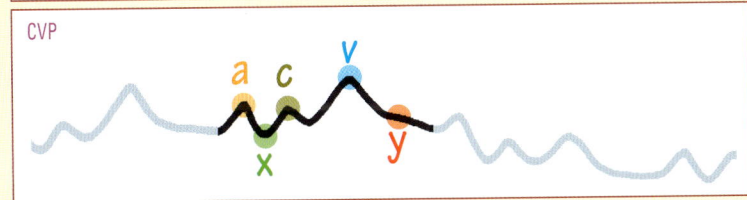

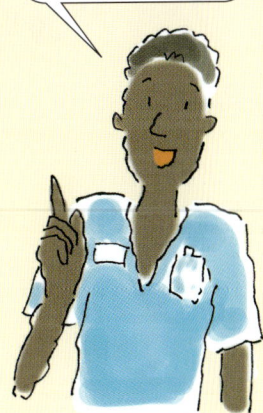

Synchronizing the CVP waveform with the ECG helps identify components. Keep in mind that cardiac electrical activity precedes systole and diastole.

Abnormal CVP waveforms

Elevated a wave

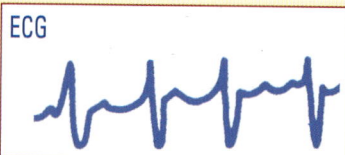

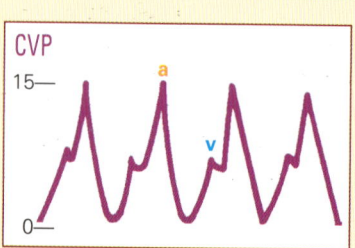

Physiologic causes
- Increased resistance to ventricular filling
- Increased atrial contraction

Associated conditions
- Heart failure
- Tricuspid stenosis
- Pulmonary hypertension

Elevated v wave

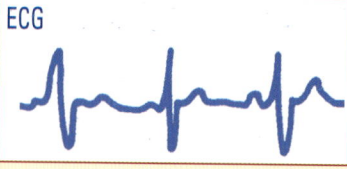

Physiologic cause
- Regurgitant flow such as in mitral regurgitation

Associated conditions
- Tricuspid insufficiency/regurgitation
- Inadequate closure of the tricuspid valve due to heart failure

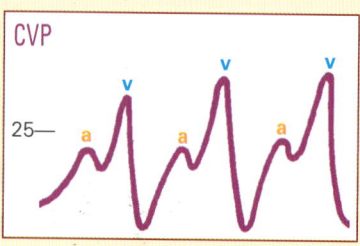

Elevated a and v waves

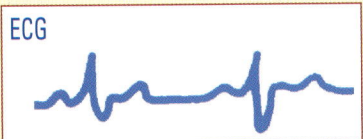

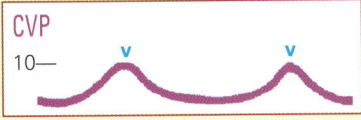

Physiologic causes
- Increased resistance to ventricular filling, which causes an elevated **a** wave
- Functional regurgitation, which causes an elevated **v** wave

Associated conditions
- Cardiac tamponade (smaller **y** descent than **x** descent)
- Constrictive pericardial disease (**y** descent exceeds **x** descent)
- Heart failure
- Hypervolemia
- Atrial hypertrophy

Absent a wave

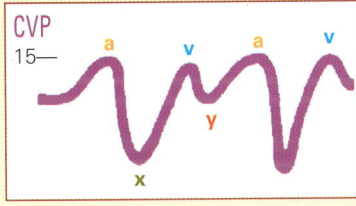

OR

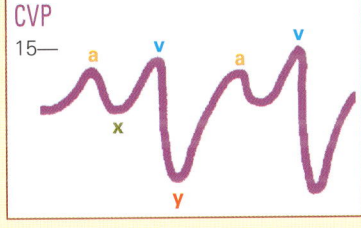

Physiologic cause
- Decreased or absent atrial contraction

Associated conditions
- Atrial fibrillation
- Junctional arrhythmias
- Ventricular pacing

Understanding CVP

CVP or right atrial pressure shows right ventricular function and end-diastolic pressure.

Causes of increased and decreased CVP

The following figure shows causes of increased pressure, normal values, and causes of decreased pressure.

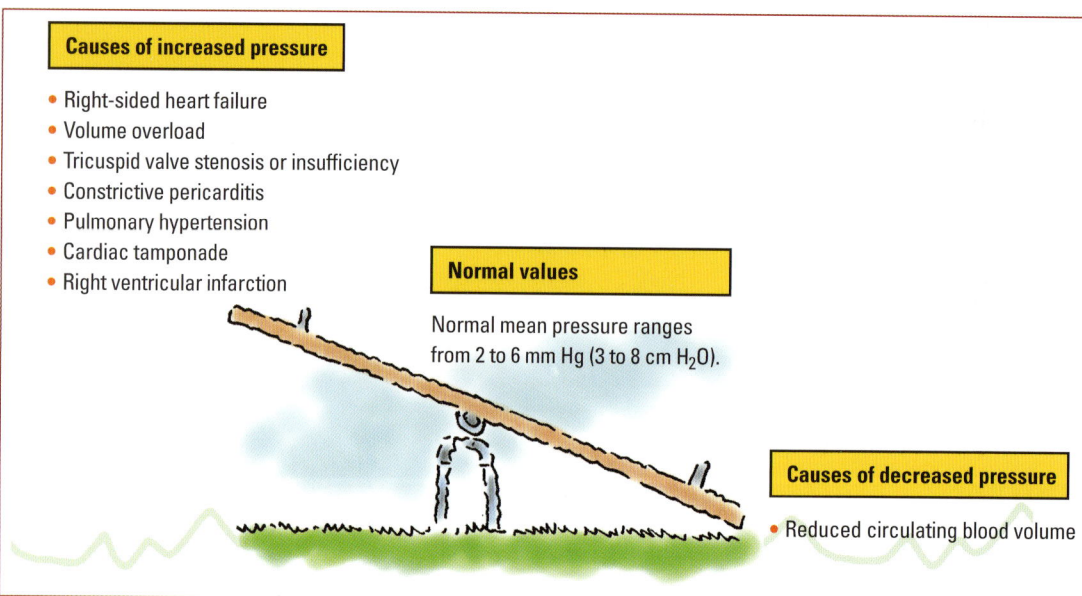

Causes of increased pressure

- Right-sided heart failure
- Volume overload
- Tricuspid valve stenosis or insufficiency
- Constrictive pericarditis
- Pulmonary hypertension
- Cardiac tamponade
- Right ventricular infarction

Normal values

Normal mean pressure ranges from 2 to 6 mm Hg (3 to 8 cm H_2O).

Causes of decreased pressure

- Reduced circulating blood volume

Key points of CVP

- The importance of CVP is that it indicates how the heart is interacting with the return of blood to the heart.
- The CVP value just before the onset of systole is an indication of the preload of the right heart.
- Normal CVP is very low.
- Under normal conditions, preload is not a major determinant of cardiac output but rather serves to provide fine-tuning of cardiac output.
- CVP values should not be used in isolation but rather in the context of the clinical situation and, preferably, with a measure of cardiac output.

(Bullet points reprinted with permission from Magder, S. (2015, October). Understanding central venous pressure: Not a preload index? *Current Opinion in Critical Care, 21*(5), 369–375. https://doi.org/10.1097/MCC.0000000000000238, Wolters Kluwer.)

Measuring CVP with a water manometer

To obtain accurate CVP readings, ensure that the manometer base is aligned with the patient's right atrium (the zero reference point). The manometer set usually contains a leveling rod to allow you to determine this alignment quickly.

After adjusting the manometer's position, examine the three-way stopcock. By turning it to any position shown in the figure that follows, you can control the direction of fluid flow. Four-way stopcocks are also available.

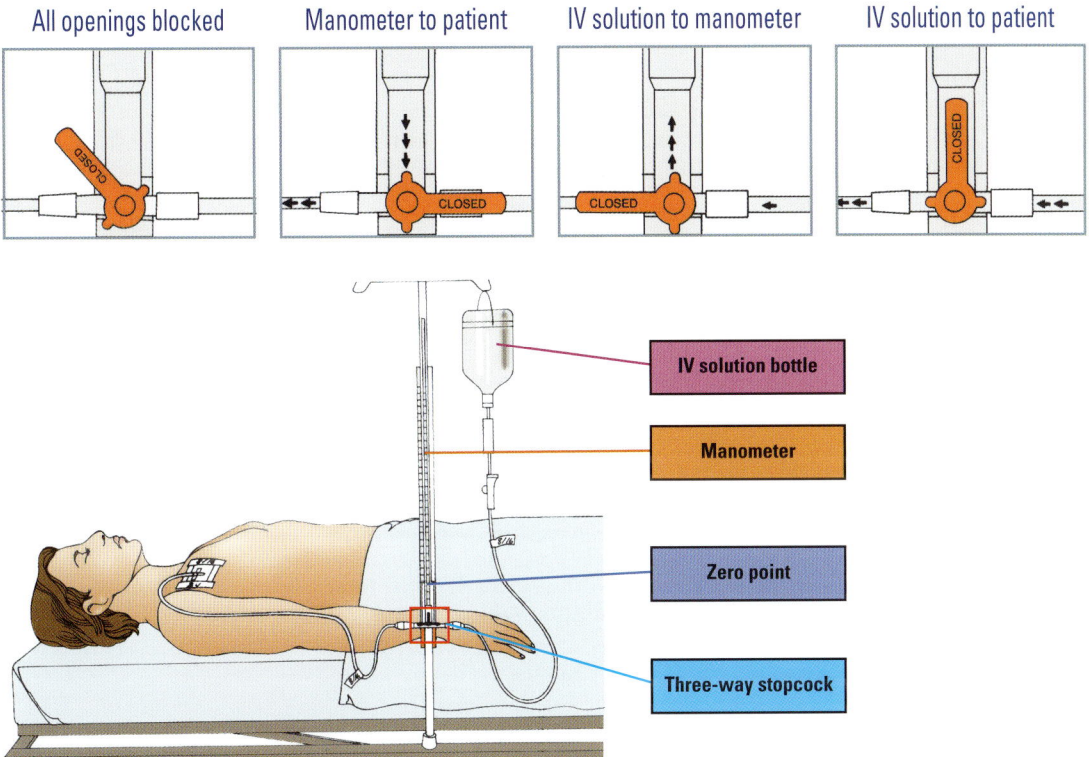

| All openings blocked | Manometer to patient | IV solution to manometer | IV solution to patient |

IV solution bottle

Manometer

Zero point

Three-way stopcock

Converting pressure values

Although most facilities today use the pressure transducer system to measure CVP, the water manometer—the first device developed for monitoring CVP—may still be in use in some facilities. Both methods measure right atrial pressure—the pressure transducer in mm Hg and the water manometer in cm H_2O. If your facility uses both pressure transducers and water manometers, you may have to convert pressure values. Use this formula to convert cm H_2O to mm Hg:

$$cm\,H_2O \div 1.36 = mm\,Hg$$

Conversely, use this formula to change mm Hg to cm H_2O:

$$mm\,Hg \times 1.36 = mm\,H_2O$$

Minimizing complications of CVP monitoring

Be on the lookout for complications that may arise, and reference the following table for troubleshooting tips.

Problem	Signs and symptoms	Possible causes
Infection	• Redness, warmth, tenderness, swelling at the insertion or exit site • Possible exudate of purulent material • Local rash or pustules • Fever, chills, malaise • Leukocytosis	• Failure to maintain sterile technique during catheter insertion or care • Wet or soiled dressing remaining on site • Immunosuppression • Contaminated catheter or solution • Frequent opening of the catheter or long-term use of a single IV access site • Failure to use good antiseptic technique when accessing the IV port
Pneumothorax, hemothorax, chylothorax, hydrothorax	• Decreased breath sounds on the affected side • With hemothorax, decreased hemoglobin level because of blood pooling • Abnormal chest x-ray	• Repeated or long-term use of the same vein • Preexisting cardiovascular disease • Lung puncture by catheter during insertion or during exchange over a guide wire • Large blood vessel puncture with bleeding inside or outside the lung • Lymph node puncture with leakage of lymph fluid • Infusion of solution into chest area through an infiltrated catheter
Air embolism	• Respiratory distress • Unequal breath sounds • Weak pulse • Increased CVP • Decreased blood pressure • Alteration or loss of consciousness	• Intake of air into the CV system during catheter insertion or tubing changes, or inadvertent opening, cutting, or breaking of catheter
Thrombosis	• Edema at puncture site • Erythema • Ipsilateral swelling of arm, neck, and face • Pain along vein • Fever, malaise • Chest pain • Dyspnea • Cyanosis	• Sluggish flow rate • Composition of catheter material (polyvinyl chloride [PVC] catheters are more thrombogenic) • Hypercoagulable state of patient (conditions like cancer, pregnancy, liver failure) • Preexisting limb edema • Infusion of irritating solutions

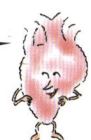

Many complications of CVP monitoring can be minimized with the right nursing interventions.

Nursing interventions	Prevention
• Monitor vital signs closely. • Re-dress the site using sterile technique. • Use a chlorhexidine-impregnated sponge at the insertion site. • Treat systemically with antibiotics or antifungals, depending on culture results. • Catheter may be removed. • Draw central and peripheral blood cultures; if the same organism appears in both, then the catheter is the primary source and should be removed. • If cultures do not match but are positive, the catheter may be removed or the infection may be treated through the catheter. • If the catheter is removed, culture its tip per facility policy. • Document interventions.	• Maintain sterile technique. Use sterile gloves, masks, and gowns when appropriate. • Clean the port per facility policy before injecting or withdrawing. • Observe dressing-change protocols. • Change a wet or soiled dressing immediately. • Change the dressing more frequently if catheter is located in femoral area or near tracheostomy. Perform tracheostomy care after catheter care. • Examine solution for cloudiness and turbidity before infusing; check the fluid container for leaks. • The catheter may be changed frequently. • Keep the system closed as much as possible.
• Notify the physician/provider. • Remove the catheter or assist with its removal. • Administer oxygen as ordered. • Set up and assist with chest tube insertion. • Document interventions.	• Position the patient head down with a rolled towel between the scapulae to dilate and expose the internal jugular or subclavian vein as much as possible during catheter insertion. • Assess for early signs of fluid infiltration (swelling in the shoulder, neck, chest, and arm). • Make sure that the patient is immobilized and prepared for insertion. An active patient may need to be sedated or taken to the operating room or interventional radiology.
• Clamp the catheter immediately. • Turn the patient on the left side, head down, so that air can enter the right atrium. Maintain this position for 20–30 minutes. • Avoid Valsalva maneuver because a large air intake worsens the condition. • Administer oxygen. • Notify the physician/provider. • Document interventions.	• Purge all air from the tubing before hookup. • Teach the patient to perform the Valsalva maneuver during catheter insertion and tubing changes. • Use air-eliminating filters. • Use an infusion pump with air detection capability. • Use Luer-lock tubing or use locking devices for all connections.
• Notify the physician/provider. • Possibly remove the catheter. • Consider treatment with anticoagulation or thrombolysis. • Verify thrombosis with diagnostic studies. • Apply warm, wet compresses locally. • Do not use the limb on the affected side for subsequent venipuncture or blood pressure measurement. • Document interventions.	• Maintain a steady flow rate with the infusion pump, or flush the catheter at regular intervals. • Use catheters made of less thrombogenic materials or catheters coated to prevent thrombosis. • Dilute irritating solutions. • Use a 0.22 micron filter for infusions.

Quick quiz

Show and tell

Identify the CV catheter insertion site in each illustration.

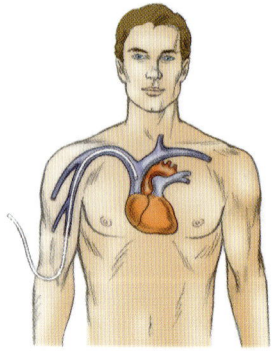 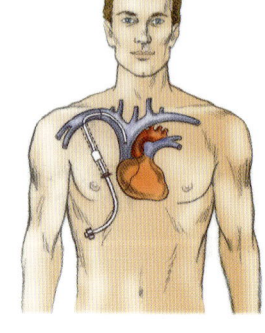 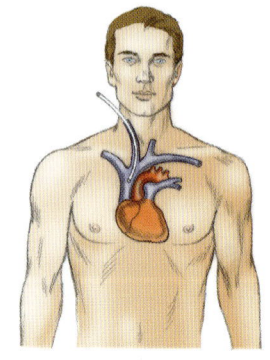

1._____   2._____   3._____

Matchmaker

Match the abnormal CVP waveforms in column 2 to their descriptions in column 1.

1. elevated **a** waves _____

A.

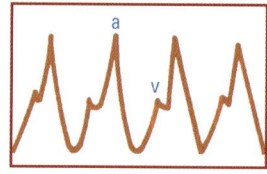

2. absent **a** waves _____

B.

3. elevated **v** waves _____

C.

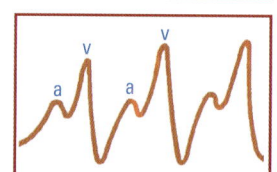

4. elevated **a** and **v** waves _____

D.

Answers: Show and tell: 1. Basilic vein; 2. Subclavian vein; 3. Internal jugular vein; Matchmaker: 1. C, 2. B, 3. D, 4. A

Selected references

Delgado, S. (2023). *AACN essentials of critical care nursing* (5th ed.). McGraw-Hill.

Diepenbrock, N. (2020). *Quick reference to critical care* (6th ed.). Lippincott Williams & Wilkins.

Hartjes, T. (Ed.). (2022). *Core curriculum for high acuity, progressive and critical care nursing* (8th ed.). W.B. Saunders Co.

Lippincott, Williams and Wilkins. (2022). *Lippincott nursing procedures* (9th ed.). Author.

McLaughlin, M. A. (2025). *Cardiovascular care made incredibly easy* (5th ed.). Wolters Kluwer.

Selby, L., Rupp, M., & Cawcutt, K. (2021). Prevention of central line–associated bloodstream infections. *Infectious Disease Clinics of North America*, 35(4), 841–856. https://doi.org/10.1016/j.idc.2021.07.004

Chapter 6

Pulmonary artery pressure monitoring

Continuous pulmonary artery pressure (PAP) and intermittent pulmonary artery wedge pressure (PAWP) measurements provide important information about left ventricular function and preload.

The components of a pulmonary artery catheter

The original PAP monitoring catheter, called a *Swan-Ganz catheter* or, more commonly, a *pulmonary artery (PA) catheter,* had two lumens. Current versions have up to six lumens, allowing for more hemodynamic information to be gathered.

In addition to distal and proximal lumens used to measure pressures, a PA catheter has a balloon inflation lumen that inflates the balloon for PAWP measurement and a thermistor connector lumen that enables cardiac output measurement. Some catheters also have a lumen that provides a port for a temporary pacemaker wire. Others have fiberoptic bundles that continuously measure mixed venous oxygen saturation.

A PA catheter is made up of the components shown in the below figure (as described on the next page):

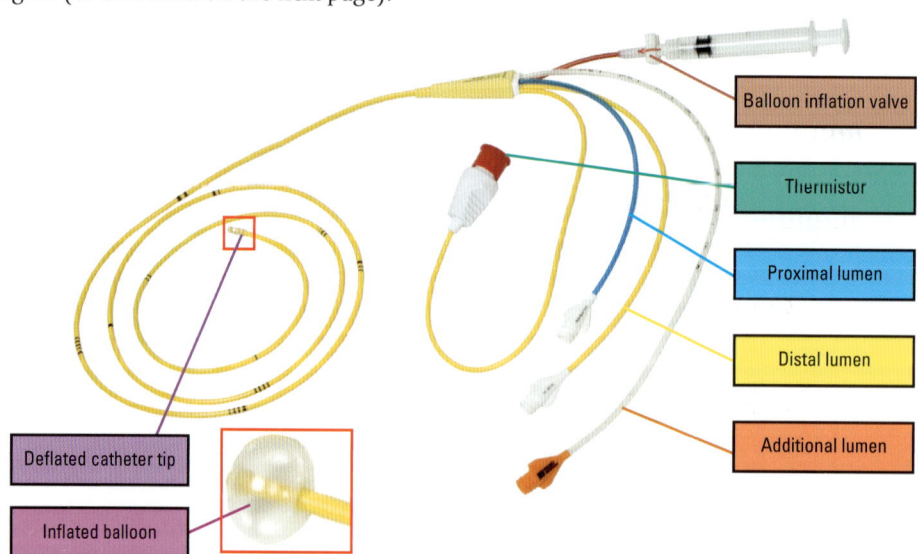

Balloon inflation valve

Thermistor

Proximal lumen

Distal lumen

Additional lumen

Deflated catheter tip

Inflated balloon

- **Deflated catheter tip:** The deflated catheter tip rests in the PA, allowing diastolic and systolic PAP readings.
- **Inflated balloon:** When inflated, the balloon wedges in a branch of the PA, allowing for PAWP measurement.
- **Balloon inflation valve:** The balloon inflation valve serves as the access point for inflating the balloon at the distal tip of the catheter for PAWP measurement.
- **Thermistor:** The thermistor measures core body temperature. When connected to a cardiac output monitor, it measures temperature changes related to cardiac output.
- **Proximal lumen:** The proximal lumen, usually blue, typically opens into the right atrium. In addition to measuring right atrial pressure, it delivers the bolus injection that is used to measure cardiac output and functions as a fluid infusion route.
- **Distal lumen:** The distal lumen, usually yellow, opens into the PA. When attached to a transducer, it measures PAP and PAWP. This port can also be used to measure mixed venous oxygen saturation.
- **Additional lumen:** This lumen provides a port for pacemaker electrodes or infusion of medications or other IV fluids.

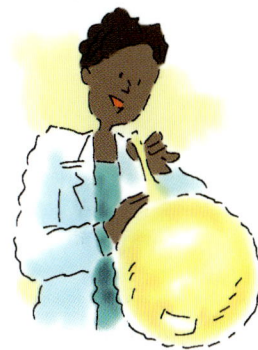

A PA catheter has a balloon inflation lumen for PAWP measurement and a thermistor connector lumen to measure cardiac output.

The components of a PAP monitoring system

Detecting pressure changes in the heart with a PA catheter involves the use of a fluid-filled monitoring system, as described in Chapter 2. The components of this system are shown in this illustration.

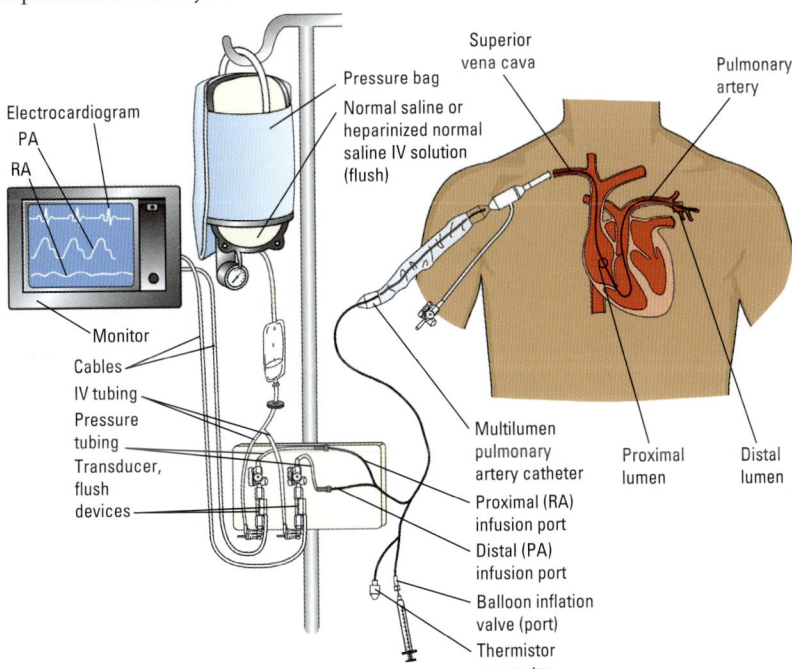

Which patients are candidates for PAP monitoring?

Nearly all patients who are acutely ill are candidates for PAP monitoring—especially those who:

- are hemodynamically unstable
- need frequent fluid or volume monitoring and management
- need continuous cardiopulmonary assessment
- are receiving multiple or frequently administered cardioactive drugs
- are in shock
- have experienced recent physical trauma
- have pulmonary, cardiac, or multisystem disease.

Cautions

Some patients require special precautions during insertion and use, including:

- those with left bundle-branch heart block
- those for whom a systemic infection would be life threatening.

Contraindications

No specific contraindications for PAP monitoring exist. However, relative contraindications include patients with:

- severe coagulation disorders
- a prosthetic right heart valve
- endocarditis
- pulmonary hypertension.

How to insert a pulmonary catheter

The balloon-tipped, multilumen catheter is inserted into the patient's internal jugular, subclavian, or femoral vein. Fluoroscopy is usually not required during catheter insertion because the catheter is flow directed, following venous blood flow from the right heart chambers into the PA. Also, the PA, right atrium, and right ventricle (RV) produce characteristic pressures and waveforms that can be observed on the monitor to help track catheter tip location. Marks on the catheter shaft, with 10-cm graduations, assist tracking by showing how far the catheter is inserted.

When the catheter reaches the right atrium, the balloon is inflated to float the catheter through the RV into the PA. PAWP measurement is then possible through an opening at the catheter's tip. The catheter (with balloon tip deflated) rests in the PA, allowing systolic and diastolic PAP readings. The balloon should be totally deflated except when taking a PAWP reading (prolonged wedging can cause pulmonary infarction).

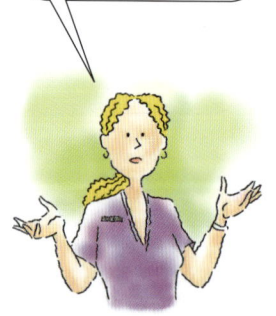

Fluoroscopy is not necessary with PA catheter insertion because the catheter follows venous blood flow into the PA!

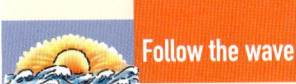

Follow the wave

Normal PA waveforms

After insertion into a large vein (usually the subclavian, jugular, or femoral vein), a PA catheter is advanced through the vena cava into the right atrium, through the RV, and into a branch of the PA. During insertion, the monitor shows various waveforms as the catheter advances through the heart chambers.

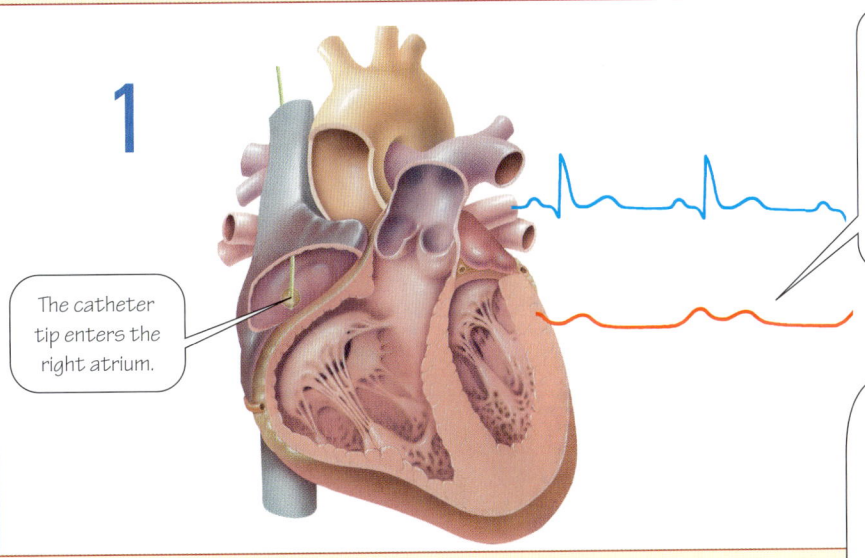

1

The catheter tip enters the right atrium.

When the catheter tip enters the right atrium, this waveform appears on the monitor, representing right atrial pressure.

Watch the patient's electrocardiogram monitor closely. Ventricular arrhythmias can occur as the catheter passes through the RV.

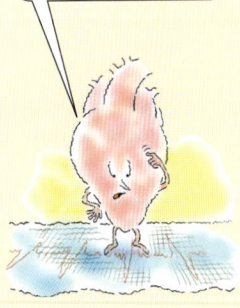

2

Next, the catheter tip reaches the right ventricle.

As the catheter tip reaches the right ventricle, you will see a waveform with sharp systolic upstrokes and lower diastolic dips.

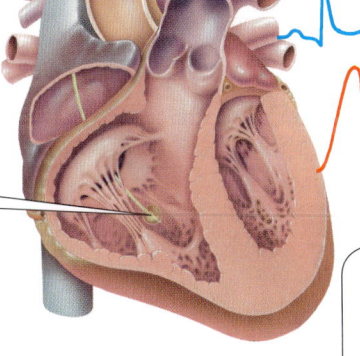

(*continued*)

Normal PA waveforms (*continued*)

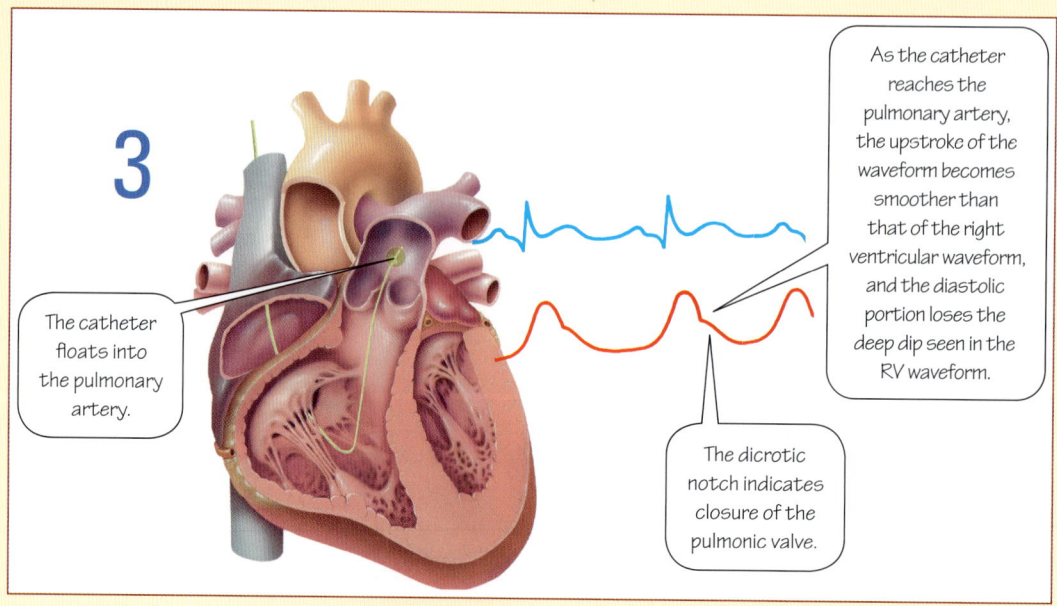

3

The catheter floats into the pulmonary artery.

As the catheter reaches the pulmonary artery, the upstroke of the waveform becomes smoother than that of the right ventricular waveform, and the diastolic portion loses the deep dip seen in the RV waveform.

The dicrotic notch indicates closure of the pulmonic valve.

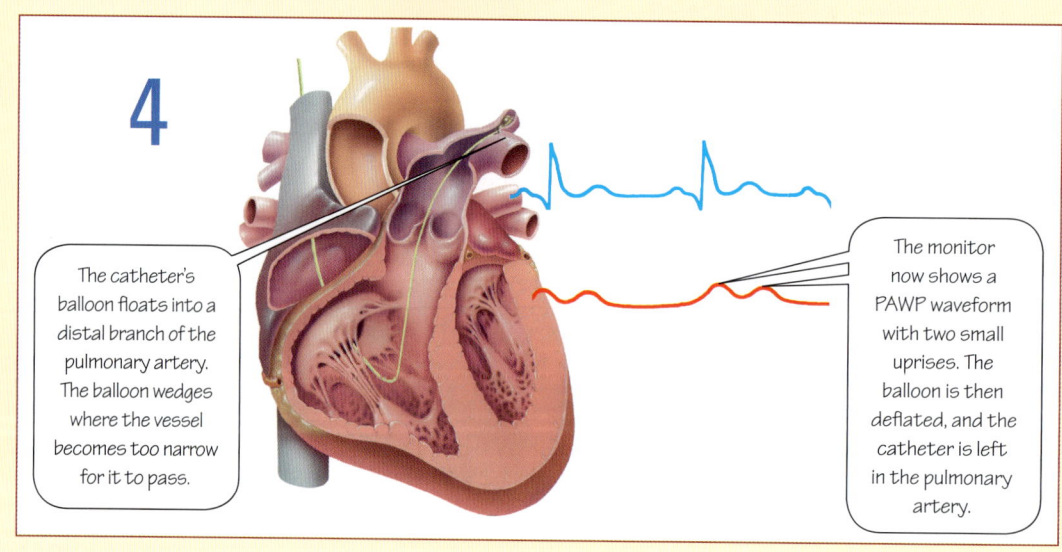

4

The catheter's balloon floats into a distal branch of the pulmonary artery. The balloon wedges where the vessel becomes too narrow for it to pass.

The monitor now shows a PAWP waveform with two small uprises. The balloon is then deflated, and the catheter is left in the pulmonary artery.

Understanding the PAP monitoring waveform

The waveform produced by PAP monitoring is similar to the arterial pressure waveform, except that the pressures are lower (because of the lower pressures in the pulmonary arteries when compared to pressures in the systemic arteries).

Follow the wave

PAP waveform

In this example of a normal PAP waveform, note that the pressure scale used is lower than the scale for arterial pressure. This waveform would be interpreted as a PAP of 32/13 mm Hg. Note that the numbers in the figure mean the following:

1. Systolic ejection into pulmonary artery
2. Closure of pulmonic valve (dicrotic notch)
3. End-diastole

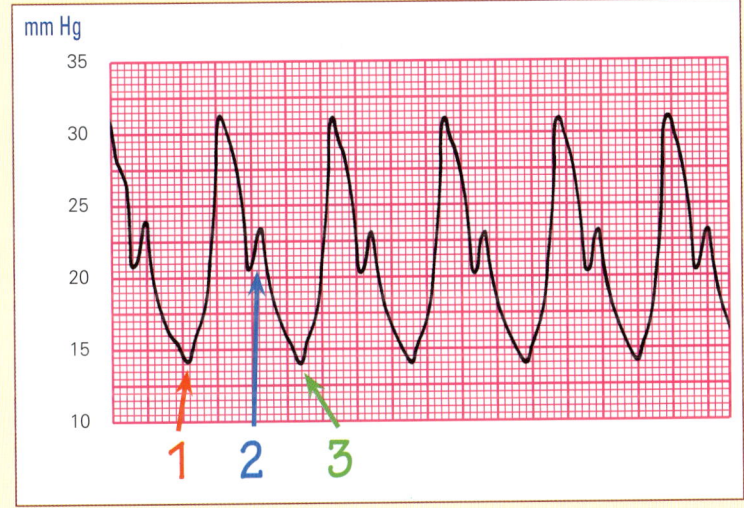

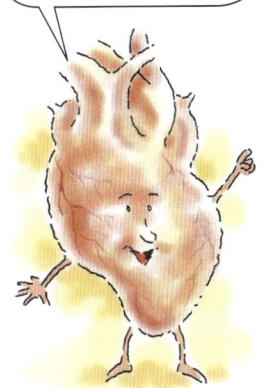

PAP monitoring records the gradients within some of my chambers and vessels.

On the level

Normal PAP parameters

PAP monitoring provides information on intracardiac pressures. To understand intracardiac pressures, picture the heart and vascular system as a continuous loop with constantly changing pressure gradients that keep blood moving. PAP monitoring records the gradients within some of the heart chambers and vessels.

(continued)

Normal PAP parameters (*continued*)

Pressure and description	Normal values	Causes of increased pressure	Causes of decreased pressure
Right ventricular pressure			
Typically, the provider measures right ventricular pressure only when initially inserting a PA catheter. Right ventricular systolic pressure normally equals PA systolic pressure. Right ventricular end-diastolic pressure reflects left ventricular function.	Normal systolic pressure ranges from 20 to 30 mm Hg; normal diastolic pressure ranges from 0 to 5 mm Hg.	• Mitral stenosis or insufficiency • Pulmonary disease • Hypoxemia • Constrictive pericarditis • Chronic heart failure • Atrial and ventricular septal defects • Patent ductus arteriosus • Pulmonary embolus	Reduced circulating blood volume
Pulmonary artery pressure			
PA systolic pressure shows right ventricular function and pulmonary circulation pressures. PA diastolic pressure reflects left ventricular pressures, specifically left ventricular end-diastolic pressure, in a patient without significant pulmonary disease.	Systolic pressure normally ranges from 20 to 30 mm Hg; normal diastolic pressure ranges from 6 to 12 mm Hg. The mean pressure usually ranges from 10 to 15 mm Hg.	• Left-sided heart failure • Increased pulmonary blood flow (left or right shunting, as in atrial or ventricular septal defects) • Any condition causing increased pulmonary arteriolar resistance, such as pulmonary hypertension, volume overload, mitral stenosis, acute respiratory distress syndrome, or hypoxia	Reduced circulating blood volume
Pulmonary artery wedge pressure			
PAWP reflects left atrial and left ventricular pressures, unless the patient has mitral stenosis. Changes in PAWP reflect changes in left ventricular filling pressure.	The mean pressure normally ranges from 4 to 12 mm Hg.	• Left-sided heart failure • Mitral stenosis or insufficiency • Pericardial tamponade	Reduced circulating blood volume

Understanding PAPs

After PA catheter insertion, PA systolic pressure and PA diastolic pressure are continuously monitored.

PAS pressure

PAS (PA systolic) pressure measures right ventricular systolic ejection or, simply put, the amount of pressure needed to open the pulmonic valve and eject blood into the pulmonary circulation. When the pulmonic valve is open, PA systolic pressure should be the same as right ventricular systolic pressure.

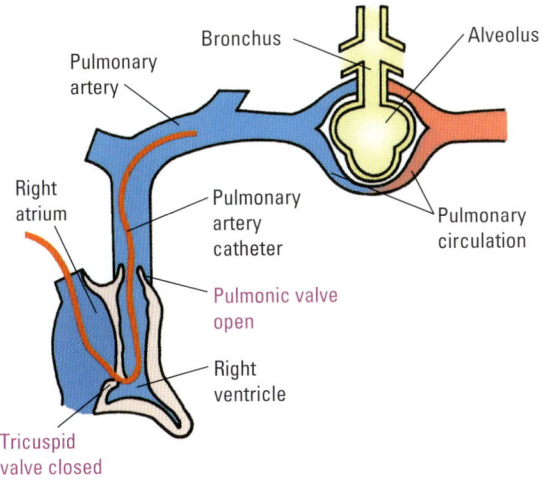

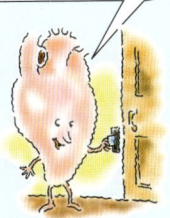

Memory jogger

To remember the difference between **PAS** and **PAD**, think of these pictures and this mnemonic.

Remember: you get a **PAS**(S) to open the door (pulmonic valve)…

PAD pressure

PAD (PA diastolic) pressure represents the resistance of the pulmonary vascular bed as measured when the pulmonic valve is closed and the mitral valve is open. To a limited degree (under absolutely normal conditions), PAD pressure also reflects left ventricular end-diastolic pressure.

…but you close the door (pulmonic valve) to your **PAD**.

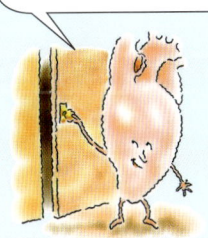

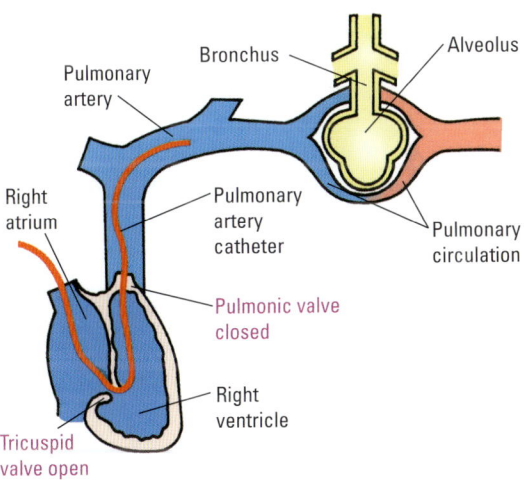

Understanding PAWP

PAWP (pulmonary artery wedge pressure) reflects left atrial and left ventricular pressures. PAWP is obtained by inflating the balloon on the PA catheter tip. The balloon floats downstream with venous blood flow to a smaller, more distal branch of the PA. Here, the catheter lodges, or wedges, causing occlusion in the forward flow of blood in the distal branch of the PA. The resulting waveform resembles that of the right atrial waveform (obtained when the balloon is deflated), except that the PAWP waveform reflects backpressure from the left side of the heart.

A closer look at the wedged position

This illustration shows the positioning of the PA catheter and its inflated tip during PAWP measurement.

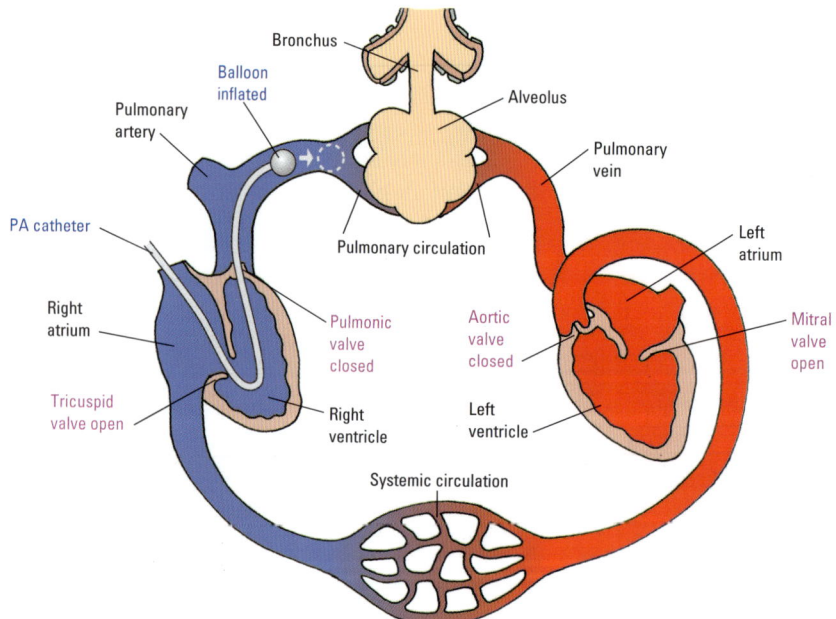

Taking a PAWP reading

By inflating the balloon and letting it float in a distal PA, you can record PAWP. Extreme caution should be used when taking a PAWP reading because of the risk of PA rupture—a rare but life-threatening complication. Know your facility's policies regarding who is permitted to obtain a PAWP reading. Make sure that you are thoroughly familiar with intracardiac waveform interpretation. Follow these steps:

1. To begin, verify that the transducer is properly leveled and zeroed. Detach the syringe from the balloon inflation hub. Draw 1.5 mL of air into the syringe, and then reattach the syringe to the hub. Watching the monitor, inject the air through the hub slowly and smoothly. When you see a wedge tracing on the monitor, immediately stop inflating the balloon. Note: Never inflate the balloon beyond the volume needed to obtain a wedge tracing; otherwise, the PA could rupture.

2. Take the pressure reading at end-expiration.

3. Note the amount of air needed to change the PA tracing to a wedge tracing (normally, 1.25 to 1.5 mL). If the wedge tracing appeared with injection of less than 1.25 mL, suspect that the catheter has migrated into a more distal branch and requires repositioning. If the balloon is in a more distal branch, the tracings may move up the oscilloscope, indicating that the catheter tip is recording balloon pressure rather than PAWP. This may lead to PA rupture.

4. Avoid prolonged wedging. Remove syringe to allow passive aspiration of the air from inflation hub. To reduce the risk of inappropriate inflation, reattach the empty syringe to the inflation hub (never reattach a syringe with air in it).

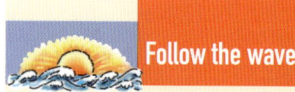

Follow the wave

Observing the PAWP waveform

On balloon inflation, you should see the normal PAP waveform flatten to the characteristic PAWP waveform. Balloon inflation should be halted on observation of this waveform. On balloon deflation, the PAP waveform should immediately reappear. Always allow the balloon to deflate passively. Actively aspirating the air in the balloon can cause balloon rupture.

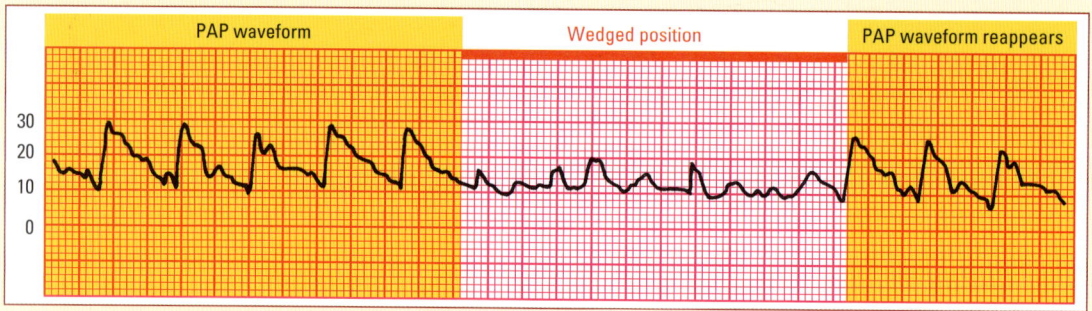

Overwedging

Prolonged wedging or hyperinflation of the balloon can produce falsely elevated PAWP measurements that are useless. Prolonged wedging or hyperinflation creates occlusion of the catheter tip and distorts accurate measurements by either:

- lodging the sensing tip of the catheter into the vessel wall, causing measurement of the pressure within the occluded catheter and high-pressure flush system
- causing the inflated balloon tip to become compressed by the surrounding PA, placing pressure on the sensing tip of the catheter.

Gently now

If an overwedging waveform is noted, gently deflate the balloon tip. The PAP waveform should reappear. Then, rewedge with less air, and avoid prolonged wedging.

> Overwedging is visible in a PAWP waveform that continuously rises or declines abruptly and then abruptly rises again.

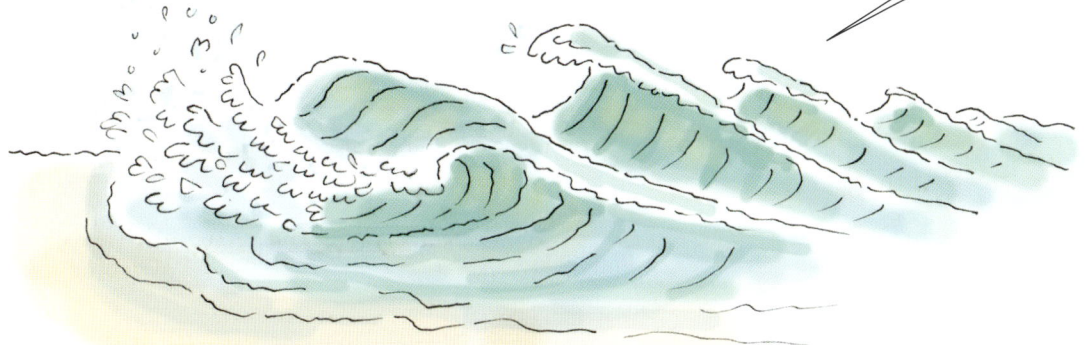

Follow the wave

Observing an overwedged waveform

The following is an example of an overwedged waveform.

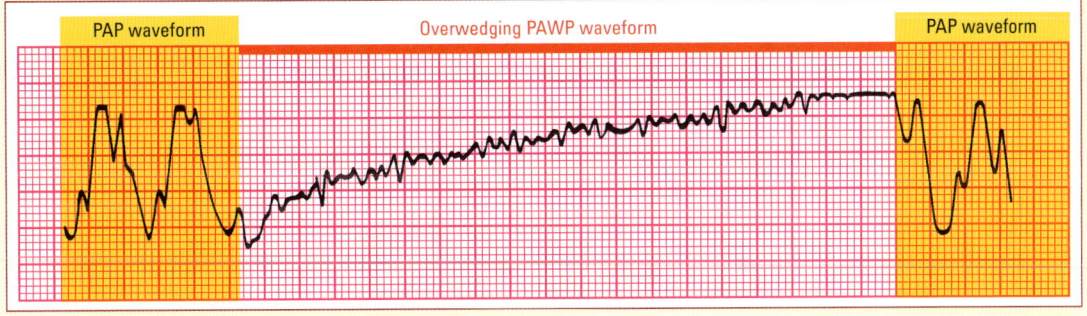

PAP waveform | Overwedging PAWP waveform | PAP waveform

Influence of intrathoracic pressure

Because the blood vessels and heart are pliable and compressible, the respiratory pressure changes that occur within the thorax may influence hemodynamic measurements. If possible, obtain PAP and PAWP values at end-expiration (when the patient completely exhales). At that time, intrathoracic pressure approaches atmospheric pressure and has the least effect on hemodynamic measurements.

If you obtain a reading during other phases of the respiratory cycle, respiratory interference may occur. For instance, during inspiration, when intrathoracic pressure drops, PAP may be false-low because the negative pressure is transmitted to the catheter. During expiration, when intrathoracic pressure rises, PAP may be false-high.

Follow the wave

Ventilatory effects on PAP and PAWP values

These waveforms illustrate how cyclical respiratory pressure changes affect PAP and PAWP measurements and highlight end-expiration points (the optimal time to obtain a reading).

Spontaneous breathing
Normal, unlabored, spontaneous respirations have a minimal effect on PAP and PAWP values, as shown below.

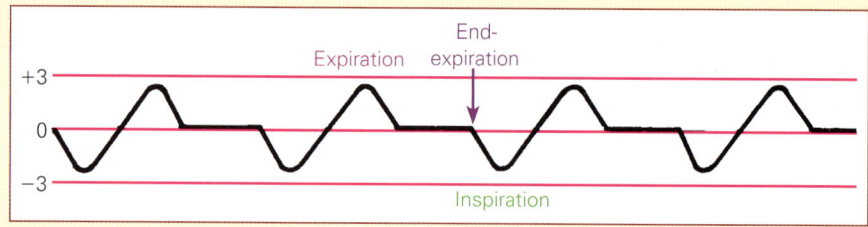

Electrocardiogram

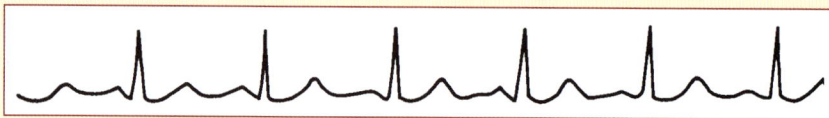

PAWP

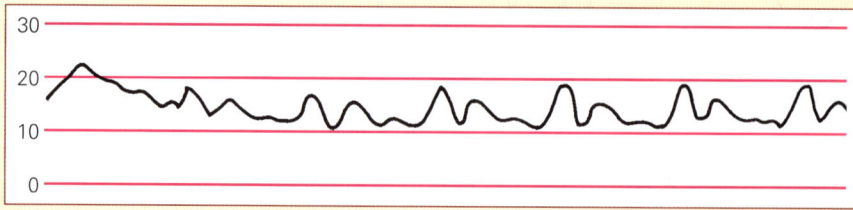

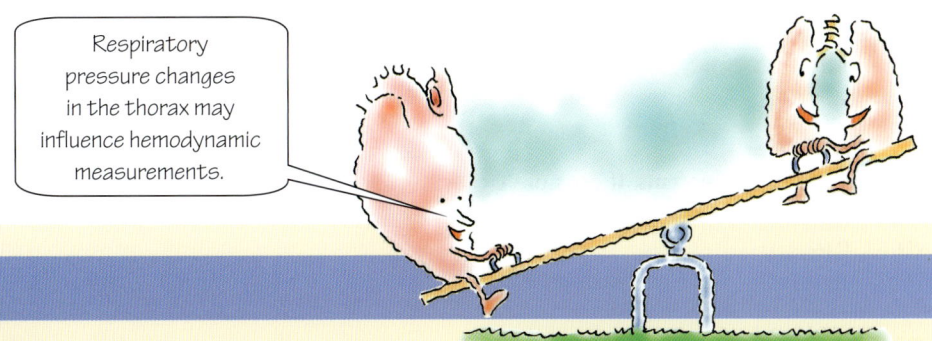

Respiratory pressure changes in the thorax may influence hemodynamic measurements.

Mechanical ventilation

When a patient is mechanically ventilated, their PAP and PAWP waveforms will follow the intrathoracic pressure changes that occur on delivery of ventilator breaths. Breaths delivered by a ventilator cause an increase in intrathoracic pressure during inspiration, the opposite of the pressure changes with spontaneous breaths. The below figures illustrate the effects of control mode ventilation, in which the ventilator delivers a preset tidal volume at a fixed rate, and synchronized intermittent mandatory ventilation (SIMV), in which the ventilator delivers a preset number of breaths at a specific tidal volume, but the patient may supplement these mechanical ventilations with their own breaths. The PAWP waveform baseline shows a combination of machine breaths and spontaneous breaths when the patient is ventilated using SIMV.

Control mode

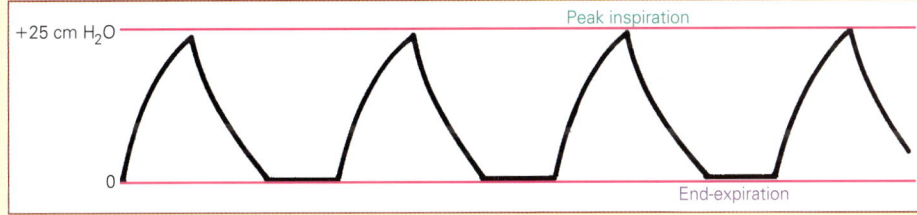

PAWP

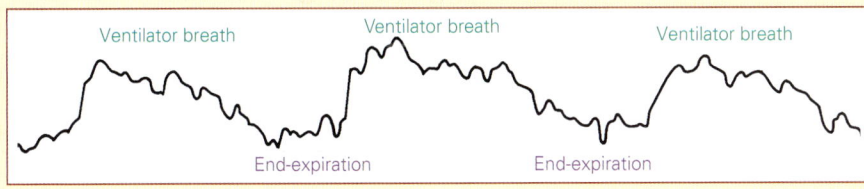

SIMV

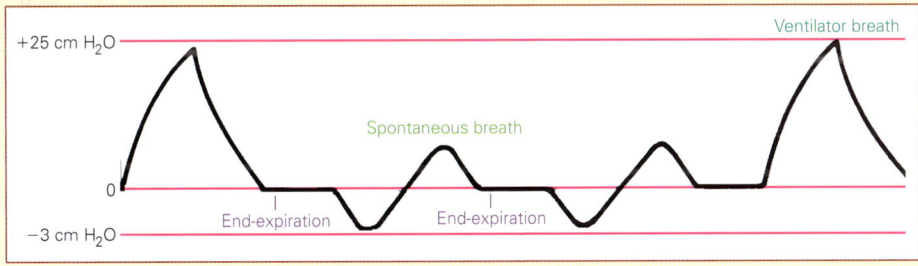

The nurse's role in PAP monitoring

Basic responsibilities

The table that follows describes the basic responsibilities of the nurse when monitoring PAP.

Responsibility	Nursing interventions
Maintain the monitoring system	• Keep the pressure on the flush bag >300 mm Hg. • Ensure that there is fluid in the flush bag. It will be depleted over time. • Keep the balloon tip deflated fully except while wedging, and keep the empty syringe attached to the inflation hub. • Never infuse medications or fluids through the PA distal lumen. • Continuously monitor the PA waveform.
Maintain accuracy of readings	• Prime the tubing and transducer carefully to avoid or remove air bubbles in the system. • Ensure the correct pressure scales on the monitor are used. • Level and zero the transducers every shift and with position changes. • Obtain pressures at end-expiration. • Inflate the balloon tip only long enough to get the wedge reading. • Use only the syringe provided with the PA catheter for wedge readings. • Note the level of catheter insertion during each shift.
Prevent infection	• Ensure sterile technique with maximal barrier precautions during PA catheter insertion. • Follow your facility's policies and procedures for accessing the PA catheter lumens. • Observe the insertion site for redness, swelling, or other signs of infection. • Monitor patient's temperature while the catheter is in place.
Educate patients and their family	• Inform the patient and their family of the purpose of the PA catheter and the rationale for using. • Let family members know how they can safely interact with the patient to avoid accidental dislodging of the PA catheter.

Minimizing complications

A patient who has a PA catheter in place is at risk for several complications. In addition to observing the patient's electrocardiogram and PAP waveform pattern and values on the bedside monitor, watch for these signs and symptoms of complications. Implement appropriate care measures to resolve or prevent them.

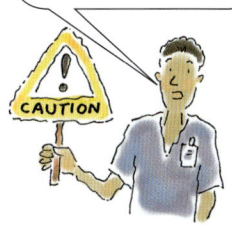

Watch for these signs and symptoms of complications from PAP monitoring.

Complications and causes	Signs and symptoms	Prevention
Bacteremia • Introduction of bacteria into the circulatory system	• Fever • Chills • Warm skin • Headache • Malaise	• Maintain strict sterile technique. • Maintain and change the monitoring setup according to facility policy.
Bleedback • Leaks in the PA catheter apparatus • Pressure bag that is inflated below 300 mm Hg	• Blood easily seen in the pressure tubing	• Tighten all connections in the monitoring setup. • Return stopcocks to their proper position after use. • Keep the pressure bag adequately inflated.
Bleeding at the insertion site • Inadequate application of pressure during and after catheter withdrawal	• Prolonged oozing or frank bleeding at the insertion site after catheter withdrawal	• Maintain pressure on the site during catheter withdrawal and for at least 10 minutes afterward. • Apply a pressure dressing over the site. • At a femoral site, apply a sandbag for 1–2 hours. • Be sure to assess distal circulation routinely, if using a sandbag, to ensure that a hematoma is not obstructing blood flow.
Pulmonary embolism • Thrombus migration from the catheter into pulmonary circulation • Clotted catheter tip from inadequate flushing	• Sharp, stabbing chest pain • Anxiety • Cyanosis • Dyspnea • Tachypnea • Diaphoresis	• Notify the provider immediately. • Administer anticoagulants as ordered. • Use a continuous flush system. • If clotting of the catheter is suspected, gently aspirate blood (with clots), and then gently irrigate the line with flush solution.
Pulmonary infarction • Catheter migration into a wedged position in the blood vessel	• Chest pain • Hemoptysis • Fever • Pleural friction rub • Low arterial oxygen levels	• Notify the provider immediately. • Never allow the balloon to be inflated for more than two respiratory cycles or 15 seconds. • After wedging, make sure a clearly defined PA waveform returns on the monitor.
Ruptured pulmonary artery • Pulmonary hypertension • Thrombus • Catheter migration into a peripheral branch of the artery • Improper inflation or prolonged wedging of the catheter's balloon	• Restlessness • Tachycardia • Hypotension • Hemoptysis • Dyspnea	• Notify the provider immediately. • Slowly inflate the balloon only until the PAWP waveform appears on the monitor, and then let the balloon deflate passively. • Never overinflate the balloon. • Reposition a migrating catheter, if permitted.

Troubleshooting

When your patient has a PA catheter, do you know how to respond to an uncharacteristic waveform on the monitor? For example, what action should you take for an erratic waveform? How should you respond to a concurrent arrhythmia on the electrocardiogram? How can you deal with an obviously inaccurate pressure reading? You should assess the patient to determine if there is an external issue, such as hypotension, causing an overdampening of the waveform. Use the chart that follows to help you recognize and resolve common problems.

Problem	Causes	Nursing interventions
No waveform on monitor	• Transducer not open to catheter • Transducer or monitor set up improperly • Defective or cracked transducer • Clotted catheter tip • Large leak in the system; loose connections	• Check the stopcock, calibration, and scale mechanisms of the system. • Tighten all connections. • Rezero the setup. • Replace the transducer.
Overdamped waveform	• Air bubbles or blood clots within the catheter or tubing • Catheter tip lodged in the vessel wall • Kinked or knotted catheter or tubing • Small leak in the system due to a loose connection	• Remove air bubbles observed in the catheter tubing and transducer. • Restore patency to a clotted catheter by gently aspirating the clot with a syringe. (Note: Never irrigate the line as a first step.) • Correct a lodged catheter by repositioning the patient or by having the patient cough and breathe deeply.
Changed waveform configuration (noisy or erratic tracings)	• Incorrectly positioned catheter • Loose connections in the setup • Faulty electrical circuitry	• Reposition the patient. • Assist with chest X-ray to verify catheter location. • Check and tighten connections in the catheter and transducer apparatus, and rezero the setup.
Ventricular irritability (paroxysmal ventricular tachycardias [PVCs] or ventricular tachycardia [V Tach])	• Irritation of the ventricular endocardium or heart valves by the catheter	• Notify the provider. (Note: The provider may prevent this problem during insertion by keeping the balloon inflated when advancing the catheter through the heart.) • Administer antiarrhythmic drugs as ordered. • Verify that the pressure waveform is not the RV waveform.
Right ventricular waveform	• Migration of the PA catheter into the right ventricle	• Notify the provider immediately. The catheter may need to be repositioned.
Catheter fling (also known as catheter motion artifact)	• Excessive catheter endovascular/intracardiac movement that may result from an arrhythmia, excessive respiratory effort, hyperdynamic circulation, excessive catheter length in the right ventricle, or location of the catheter tip near the pulmonic valve	• Notify the provider for catheter repositioning.
Falsely increased or decreased pressure readings	• System not properly leveled or zeroed • Patient's body or bed repositioned without releveling or rezeroing the system	• Reposition the transducer level with the phlebostatic axis. • Rezero the monitor.

Problem	Causes	Nursing interventions
Continuous PAWP waveform	• Catheter migration • Balloon still inflated	• Verify that the balloon is deflated. • Reposition the patient or have them cough and breathe deeply. • Notify the provider for catheter repositioning.
Missing PAWP waveform	• Malpositioned catheter • Kinked or knotted tubing • Insufficient air in the balloon tip • Ruptured balloon	• Reposition the patient, and check tubing patency. • Reinflate the balloon adequately • Assess the balloon's competence. (Note resistance during inflation, feel how the syringe's plunger springs back after the balloon inflates, and check for blood leaking from the balloon lumen.) • If the balloon has lost its competence, it has likely ruptured. Turn the patient onto their left side, tape the balloon inflation port, and notify the provider.

Quick quiz

Matchmaker

Match the PAP monitoring problem to the possible cause.

1. Overdamped waveform_____

2. Right ventricular waveform_____

3. Falsely increased or decreased pressure readings_____

4. Missing PAWP waveform_____

A. insufficient air in the balloon tip

B. migration of the PA catheter into the right ventricle

C. catheter tip lodged in the vessel wall

D. patient's body or bed repositioned without releveling or rezeroing the system

Show and tell

Identify the waveform in each illustration.

1. _____

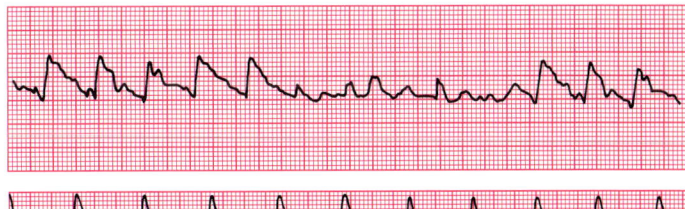

2. _____

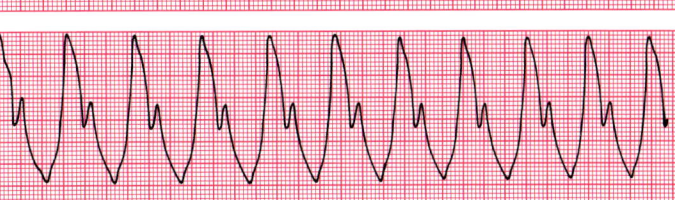

3. _____

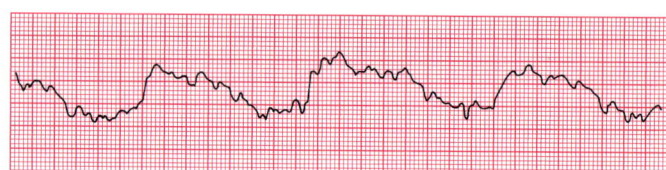

What do you know?

1. Your patient had a PA catheter placed earlier today. What would you do if you saw this waveform on the monitor?

_____

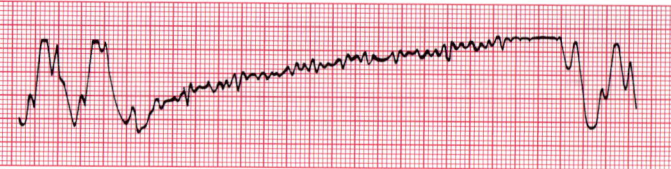

2. What is the PAWP pressure on this spontaneously breathing patient?

_____

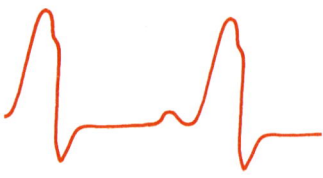

3. Which hemodynamic parameter can be used instead of the PAWP to assess left ventricular function?

_____

Answers: Matchmaker: 1. C, 2. B, 3. D, 4. A; Show and tell: 1. Normal PAWP waveform, 2. Normal PAP waveform, 3. Overwedged waveform; What do you know? 1. Notify the provider to reposition the PA catheter. The tip has migrated to the right ventricle. 2. I can determine the answer when the scale is available. 3. Pulmonary artery diastolic (PAD) pressure

---

Selected references

Centers for Disease Control and Prevention. (2023). *Guidelines for the prevention of intravascular catheter-related infections.* Retrieved June 20, 2023, from https://www.cdc.gov/infectioncontrol/guidelines/bsi/updates.html#anchor_1554127635

Delgado, S. (2023). *AACN essentials of critical care nursing* (5th ed.). McGraw-Hill.

Diepenbrock, N. (2020). *Quick reference to critical care* (6th ed.). Lippincott Williams & Wilkins.

Hartjes, T. (Ed.). (2022). *Core curriculum for high acuity, progressive and critical care nursing* (8th ed.). W.B. Saunders Co.

Johnson, K. (Ed.). (2023). *AACN procedure manual for progressive and critical care* (8th ed.). Elsevier.

Lippincott's nursing procedures & skills (9th ed.). (2022). Lippincott Williams & Wilkins.

McLaughlin, M. A. (2025). *Cardiovascular care made incredibly easy* (5th ed.). Wolters Kluwer.

Chapter 7

Cardiac output monitoring

Understanding cardiac output monitoring

Measuring cardiac output

Measuring cardiac output (CO)—the amount of blood ejected by the heart over 1 minute—helps evaluate cardiac function. CO is a function of heart rate (HR) multiplied by stroke volume (SV), and the three major components of SV are preload, afterload, and contractility. Historically, the "gold standard" for CO monitoring was invasive measurement using a thermodilution pulmonary artery catheter (PAC). PACs provide a volume of information, but they also expose the patient to specific potential complications and require care providers who maintain competence in PAC management. Newer technologies are striving to accomplish CO measurement through less invasive methodologies. Currently, CO assessment can be accomplished through noninvasive, minimally invasive, or invasive techniques. Let's briefly review the potential methodologies.

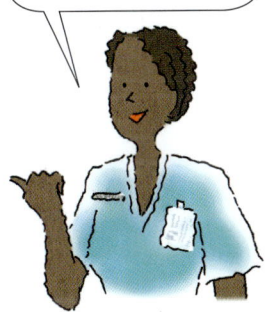

Noninvasive, minimally invasive, or invasive technologies can be used to assess CO.

Noninvasive technologies

Noninvasive techniques include bioimpedance/bioreactance, noninvasive arterial pressure waveform, and echocardiography.

Bioimpedance/bioreactance

Bioimpedance/bioreactance methodologies employ the use of several thoracic skin electrodes to calculate CO. The reliability and validity of these technologies have not been established in many patient populations, providing limited applicability in the critical care setting.

Noninvasive arterial pressure waveform

Noninvasive arterial pressure waveform uses inflatable finger cuffs along with a device to measure arterial diameter in the fingers. CO is calculated based upon the increase in arterial diameter during systole. This technology has shown varying degrees of accuracy in a variety of patient populations, so more evidence is required to determine optimal application of this technology.

Echocardiography

Echocardiography has been used diagnostically and can provide a one-time measurement of CO during testing. Limitations in obtaining continuous or repetitive measurements reduce the applicability of echocardiography in the critical care setting.

Minimally invasive technologies

Minimally invasive techniques such as invasive pulse wave analysis or esophageal Doppler provide CO measurements as well.

Invasive pulse wave analysis

Invasive pulse wave analysis requires placement of an arterial pressure monitoring catheter. This technology provides CO measurements based upon arterial waveform analysis and can also provide indicators of fluid responsiveness in certain patient populations. Arterial pressure monitoring devices are quite easy to use and are gaining popularity because many critically ill patients already have arterial pressure monitoring in place.

Esophageal Doppler

An esophageal Doppler estimates CO from blood flowing in the descending thoracic aorta based on signals obtained from a probe inserted into the patient's esophagus. This technology requires significant patient sedation to reduce gagging and to ensure correct placement of the probe. These technologies are quite useful in the perioperative setting but have more limited usefulness in the critical care setting for ongoing monitoring and measurement.

Invasive technologies

CO monitoring devices are invasive technologies; these include lithium-ion dilution, transpulmonary thermodilution coupled with pulse wave analysis, Fick method, and thermodilution PACs.

Lithium-ion dilution

Lithium-ion dilution technology requires placement of a radial arterial pressure monitoring catheter and a central venous catheter. Injections of lithium ion are accomplished through the central venous catheter. Measurement of lithium-ion concentration is accomplished through radial artery blood sampling, which then provides intermittent CO measurements. This methodology requires repeated arterial blood sampling and administration of lithium ion, both of which can create issues in the critically ill.

Transpulmonary thermodilution and pulse wave analysis

Transpulmonary thermodilution and pulse wave analysis technologies require placement of a central venous catheter as well as a specialized thermistor-tipped femoral arterial catheter. Warmed fluid boluses are delivered through the central venous catheter, and the change in temperature over time is measured by the thermistor located in the femoral artery. The temperature change over time represents CO flow from the central venous catheter to the thermistor in the femoral artery. A variety of parameters are calculated in addition to CO measurements, providing additional information for patient management. Multiple pathophysiologic conditions can impact the accuracy and applicability of this technology.

The Fick method

The Fick method is useful in estimating CO based upon arterial and venous oxygen levels and oxygen consumption. Fick CO is equal to oxygen consumption divided by the arterial-venous oxygen content difference. To calculate an estimated Fick CO, the following information is required:

- **Hemoglobin:** The most recently obtained hemoglobin level
- **Arterial oxygen content:** The combination of oxygen dissolved in the arterial blood (pO_2) and the arterial oxygen saturation (SaO_2). These values are obtained from arterial blood gas analysis. Because the pO_2 provides only a small contribution to total arterial oxygen content, calculations are frequently done using only arterial oxygen saturation. At times, if no invasive specimen can be obtained, a reliable arterial pulse oximetry value can be substituted.
- **Venous oxygen content:** The combination of oxygen dissolved in the mixed venous blood (pvO_2) and the venous oxygen saturation (SvO_2). These values are obtained from a mixed venous blood gas analysis. Similar to arterial oxygen content calculations, because the pvO_2 provides only a small contribution to total venous oxygen content, calculations are frequently done using only venous oxygen saturation. Ideally, a true mixed venous sample is obtained from the pulmonary artery (PA). If PA sampling is not available, central venous O_2 saturation can be substituted.
- **Oxygen consumption:** This is measured with a spirometer. In many cases, a standard estimated value of 125 mL/min at rest is used. Some authorities substitute 110 mL/min for patients assigned female at birth.

    Many convenient Fick calculators are available that provide an estimated CO after current patient values are entered. Fick calculation can provide a rapid estimation of CO in patients with readily available arterial and venous oxygen saturation measurements.

Thermodilution PACs

The most well-validated method for monitoring CO is the thermodilution technique, and the indicator dilution method with use of a PAC is still considered the gold standard of measurement.

Performed at the bedside, the thermodilution technique evaluates the cardiac status of critically ill patients and those suspected of having cardiac disease. This technique is the method focused on in this chapter.

On the level

What causes changes in CO?

Normally, CO ranges from 4 to 8 L/min. Values below this range may result from:
- decreased myocardial contractility caused by myocardial damage, drug effects, acidosis, or hypoxia.
- decreased filling pressure (reduced preload).
- increased systemic vascular resistance (SVR; increased afterload) related to arteriosclerosis, vasoconstriction, or hypertension.
- dysrhythmias.
- decreased ventricular flow related to valvular heart disease.
- high CO that can occur with some arteriovenous shunts and from decreased vascular resistance (as in septic shock).

In some cases, an unusually high CO can be normal—for example, in well-conditioned athletes.

Thermodilution methods

Bedside CO measurements are obtained by an intermittent bolus method or a continuous CO (CCO) method.

The intermittent bolus thermodilution method

To measure CO using the intermittent bolus thermodilution method, a quantity of solution at least 10 degrees cooler than the patient's blood is injected into the right atrium through the proximal injectate (blue) lumen on a PAC. This indicator solution mixes with the blood as it travels through the right ventricle into the PA, and a thermistor on the catheter registers the change in temperature of the flowing blood. A computer then plots the temperature change over time as a curve and calculates the flow based on the area under the curve.

A closer look at the intermittent bolus thermodilution method

The steps in the path the injectate solution takes through the heart during intermittent bolus thermodilution CO monitoring are described here and illustrated in the figure below:

1. The cold injectate is introduced into the right atrium through the proximal injection port of the PAC. The temperature of the injectate is measured as it is injected.
2. The injectate solution mixes completely with the blood in the right ventricle.
3. The cooled blood then flows into the PA, and a thermistor on the catheter registers the change in the temperature of the blood.

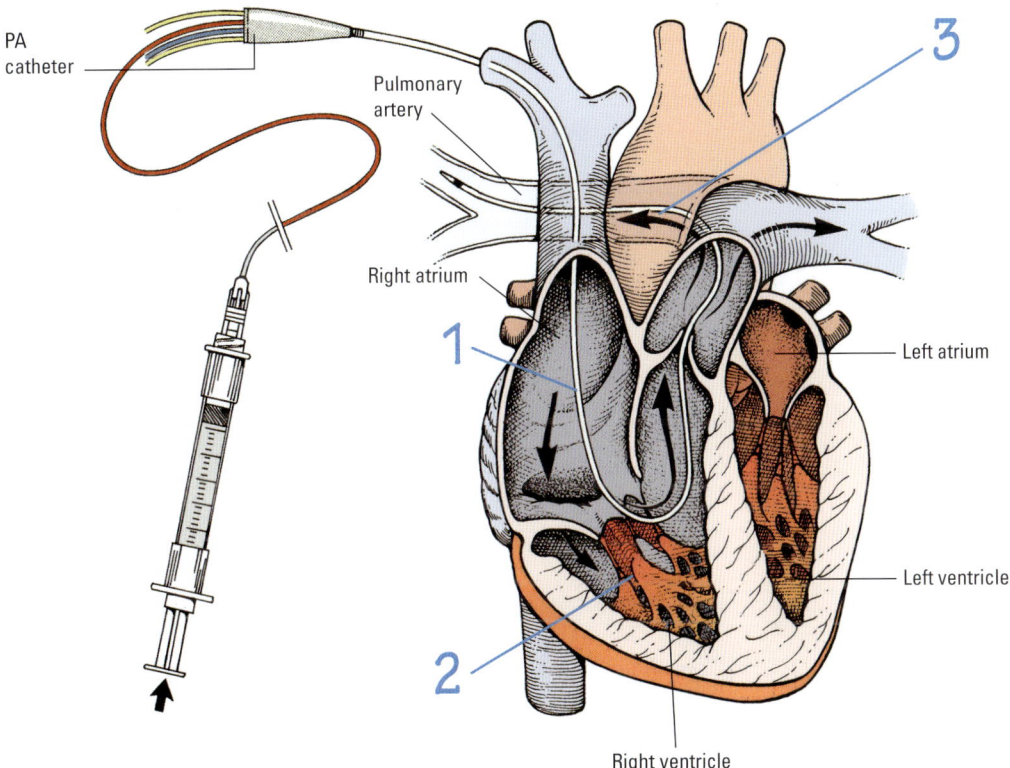

PA catheter

Pulmonary artery

Right atrium

1

2

Right ventricle

3

Left atrium

Left ventricle

Intermittent bolus thermodilution setup

Equipment and supplies used for this thermodilution method include a thermodilution PAC in the correct position, a CO computer and cables (or a module for the bedside cardiac monitor), a closed or open injectate delivery system, a 10-mL syringe, a 500-mL bag of injectate solution (typically 0.9% sodium chloride), and crushed ice and water, or cooling unit (if iced injectant is to be used).

The following illustration shows a PAC prepared for CO monitoring.

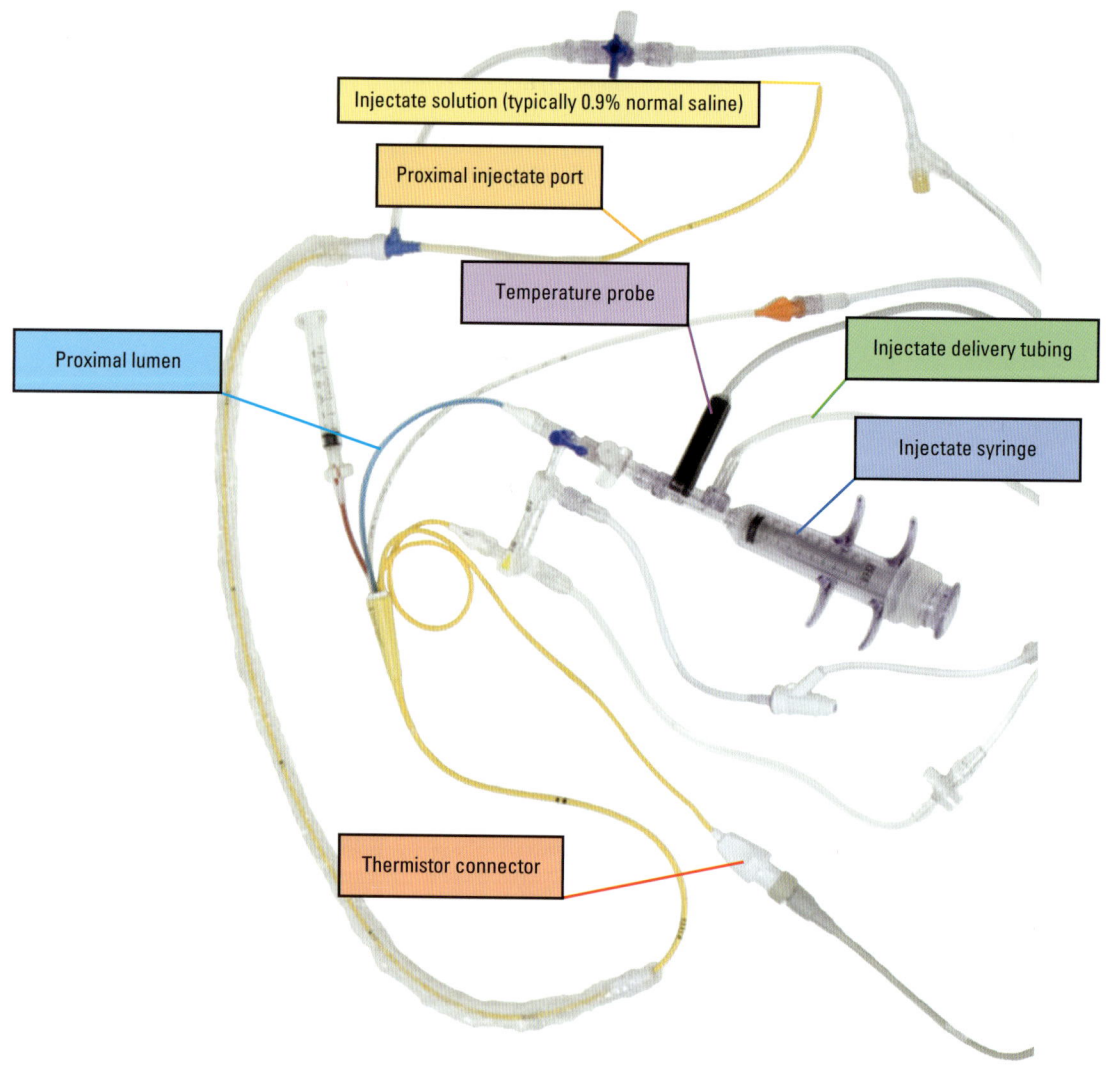

Injectate solution (typically 0.9% normal saline)

Proximal injectate port

Temperature probe

Injectate delivery tubing

Proximal lumen

Injectate syringe

Thermistor connector

The CCO method

Measuring CO using a CCO system requires an advanced PAC and a CCO computer. Rather than using a cooler-than-blood injectant as the signal, the CCO system relies on a thermal filament on the catheter's outer surface. The thermal filament creates a signal by emitting pulses of low-heat energy, warming blood as it flows by; a thermistor then measures the temperature downstream. A computer algorithm identifies when the PA temperature change matches the temperature of the signal and produces a thermodilution washout curve and the CO value.

The monitor measures CO about every 30 to 60 seconds and displays a continuously updated CO value, averaged from the previous 3 to 6 minutes of data collected. CCO technology correlates well with bolus thermodilution measurements, eliminates the need for additional fluid administration, and provides ongoing trending information.

A closer look at the CCO method

The following figure illustrates the CCO method.

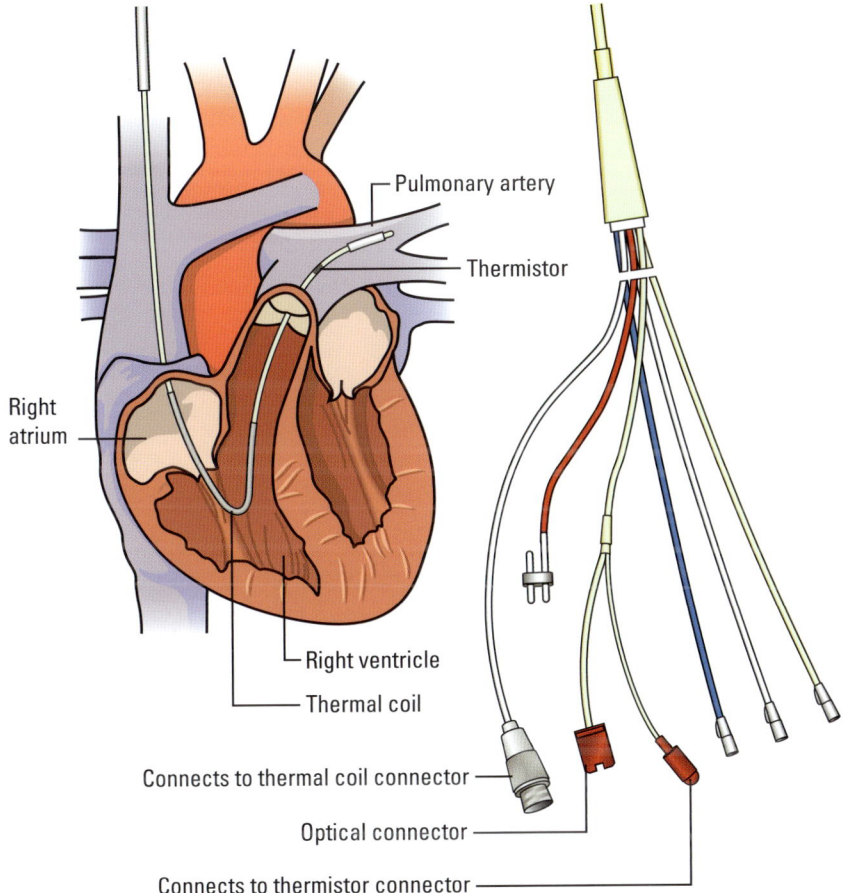

Pulmonary artery

Thermistor

Right atrium

Right ventricle

Thermal coil

Connects to thermal coil connector

Optical connector

Connects to thermistor connector

Measuring an intermittent bolus CO

Either iced or room temperature injectate may be used when measuring an intermittent bolus CO (see *Injectate temperature considerations*).

Injectate temperature considerations

Iced or room temperature injectate may be used. Consider the following when choosing which to use:
- The choice should be based on facility policy as well as the patient's status.
- The accuracy of the bolus thermodilution technique depends on the computer being able to differentiate the temperature change caused by the injectate in the PA. Because iced injectate is colder than room temperature injectate, it provides a stronger signal to be detected.
- Room temperature injectate is more convenient and provides an accurate result as long as there is at least a 10-degree difference between the injectate and blood temperatures.
- Iced injectate may be more accurate in patients with high or low CO or hypothermia or when smaller volumes of injectate must be used (3 to 5 mL), as in patients with volume restrictions or in children.
- The acceptable temperature range for iced versus room temperature injectate varies by manufacturer. Generally, room temperature is 18°C to 25°C and cold or iced injectate is 0°C to 12°C (Johnson, 2023).

Room temperature injectate with a closed delivery system

Follow these steps:
1. Position the patient in the supine position with head of bed between 0 and 20 degrees.
2. Connect the primed system to the stopcock of the proximal injectate lumen of the PAC. Consider presence of any infusions also infusing through the proximal injectate lumen. Relocate medicated infusions to alternative infusion sites.
3. Connect the temperature probe from the CO computer to the closed injectate system's flow-through housing device.
4. Connect the CO computer cable to the thermistor connector on the PAC, and verify the blood temperature reading.
5. Turn on the CO computer, and enter the correct computation constant (CC) as provided by the catheter's manufacturer. The constant is determined by the volume and temperature of the injectate as well as the size and type of catheter. Ensure that the CC is correct for the volume and temperature of the injectate that is being used.
6. Verify that the injectate temperature is at least 10 degrees cooler than the patient's blood temperature.
7. Verify the presence of central venous and PA waveforms on the cardiac monitor to verify proper position of the PAC.
8. Withdraw exactly 10 mL (or alternative volume) of injectate.
9. Turn the stopcock at the catheter injectate hub to open a fluid path between the injectate lumen of the PAC and the syringe.

10. Press the START button on the CO computer or wait for the INJECT message to display. Observe the patient's respiratory pattern, and inject the solution at end-expiration smoothly within 4 seconds, making sure that it does not leak at the connectors.

> The injection should take no longer than 4 seconds to complete.

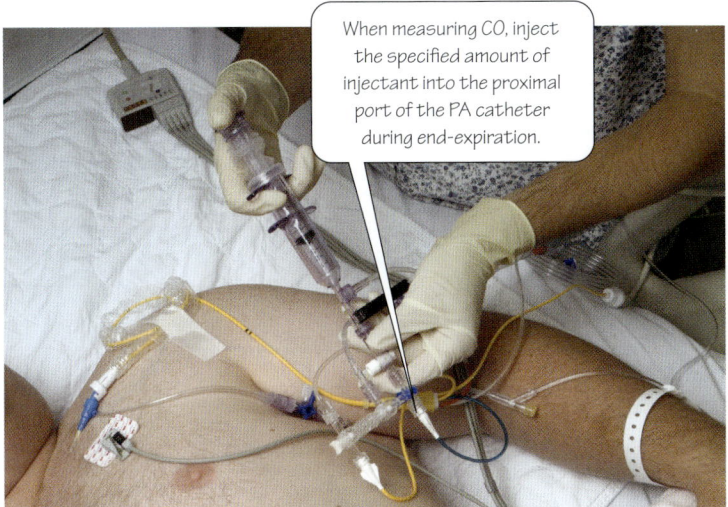

> When measuring CO, inject the specified amount of injectant into the proximal port of the PA catheter during end-expiration.

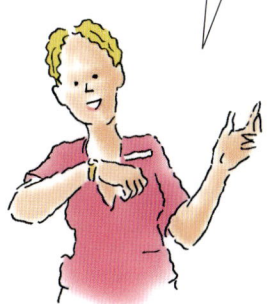

11. Analyze the contour of the thermodilution curve for a flat baseline, smooth upstroke, and a gradual downstroke. Discard abnormal curves.

12. Wait 1 to 2 minutes between injections or until the CO computer displays that it is ready for a new injection. Repeat the procedure until three values are 10% to 15% of the median value. Compute the average, and record the patient's CO.

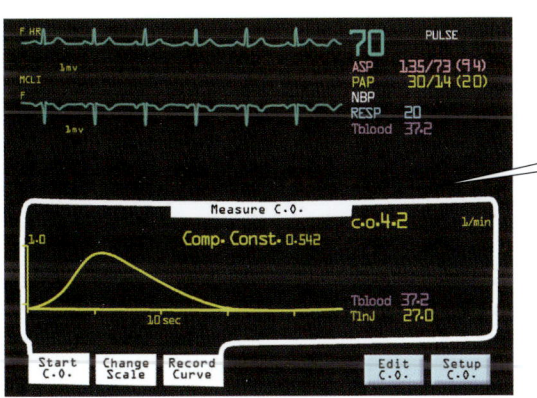

> Check the thermodilution curve on the patient's monitor to make sure that the injection was properly performed. You should see a smooth, sharp rise in the curve. Repeat the injection procedure at least 3 times to obtain a mean CO value.

13. Return the stopcock to its original position and clamp the injectate delivery system.

14. Verify the presence of central venous and PA waveforms on the cardiac monitor. Repeat bolus CO measurements every 4 hours, as ordered by the provider, or as clinically indicated.

Iced injectate with a closed delivery system

Follow these steps:

1. Place the coiled segment of the tubing into the Styrofoam container and add crushed ice and water to cover the entire coil or use a cooling unit supplied by the manufacturer.
2. Let the solution cool for 15 to 20 minutes.
3. Proceed as for the room temperature injectate with a closed delivery system.

Follow the wave

Analyzing thermodilution curves

The thermodilution curve provides valuable information about CO, injection technique, and equipment problems. When studying the curve, keep in mind that the area under the curve is inversely proportionate to CO: The smaller the area under the curve, the higher the CO; the larger the area under the curve, the lower the CO.

Besides providing a record of CO, the curve may indicate problems related to technique, such as erratic or slow injectate instillations, or other problems, such as respiratory variations or electrical interference. The curves shown here correspond to those typically seen in clinical practice.

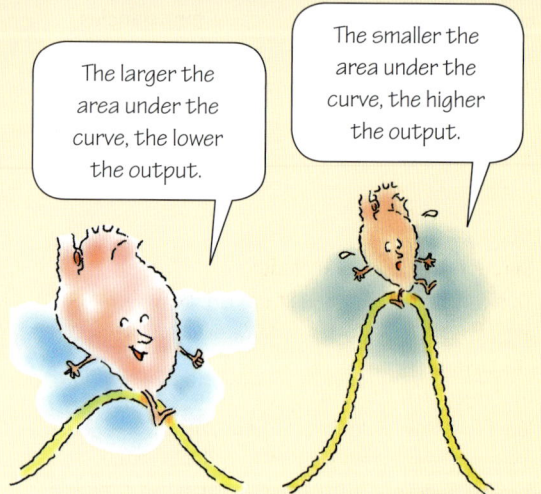

The larger the area under the curve, the lower the output.

The smaller the area under the curve, the higher the output.

Normal thermodilution curve

With an accurate monitoring system and a patient who has adequate CO, the thermodilution curve begins with a smooth, rapid upstroke and rounded peak, and is followed by a smooth, gradual downslope. The curve shown in this figure indicates that the injectate instillation time was within the recommended 4 seconds and that the temperature curve returned to baseline blood temperature.

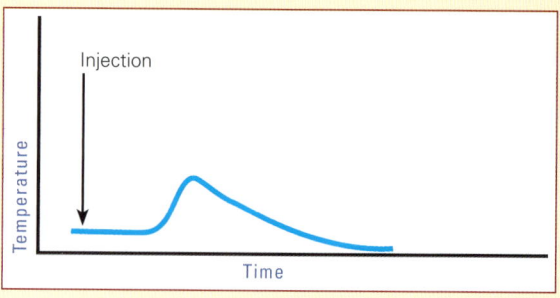

The height of the curve will vary, depending on whether you use a room temperature injectate or an iced injectate. A room temperature injectate produces an upstroke of lower amplitude.

Low CO curve

A thermodilution curve representing low CO shows a rapid, smooth upstroke (from proper injection technique). However, because the heart is ejecting blood less efficiently from the ventricles, the injectate warms slowly and takes longer to be ejected from the ventricle. Consequently, the curve takes longer to return to baseline. This slow return produces a larger area under the curve, corresponding to low CO.

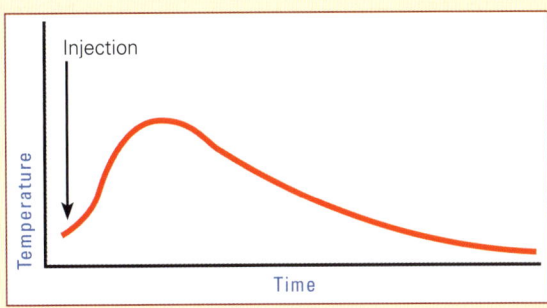

High CO curve

Again, the curve has a rapid, smooth upstroke from proper injection technique. Because the ventricles are ejecting blood forcefully or rapidly, the injectate moves through the heart quickly, and the curve returns to baseline rapidly. The smaller area under the curve suggests higher CO.

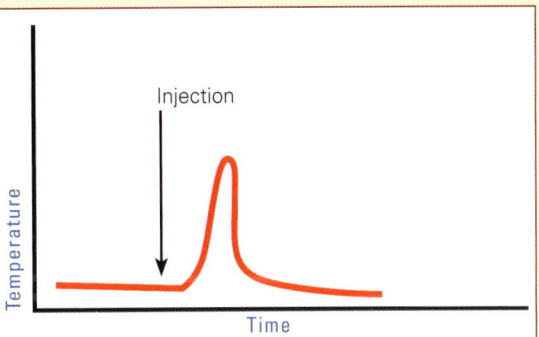

Curve reflecting poor technique

This curve results from an uneven or too slow (taking more than 4 seconds) administration of injectate. The uneven and slower-than-normal upstroke and the larger area under the curve erroneously indicate low CO. A kinked catheter, unsteady hands during the injection, or improper placement of the injectate lumen in the introducer sheath may also cause this type of curve.

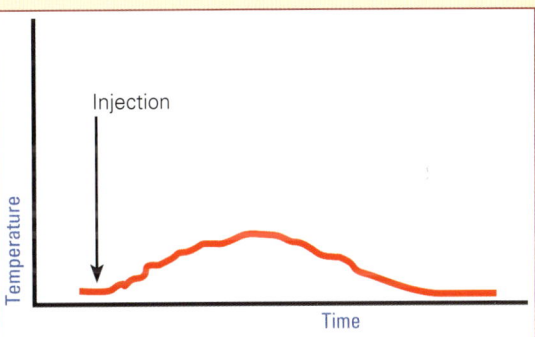

Curve associated with respiratory variations

To obtain a reliable CO measurement, a steady baseline PA blood temperature is required. If the patient has rapid or labored respirations, or is receiving mechanical ventilation, the thermodilution curve may reflect inaccurate CO values. The curve shown in this figure from a patient receiving mechanical ventilation reflects fluctuating PA blood temperatures. The thermistor interprets the unsteady temperature as a return to baseline. The result is a

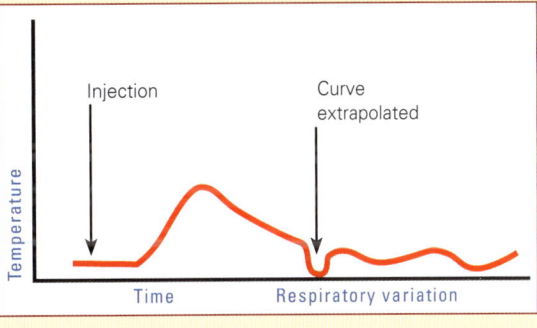

curve erroneously showing a high CO (small area under the curve). (Note: In some cases, the equipment senses no return to baseline at all and produces a sinelike curve recorded by the computer as 0.00.)

Measuring cardiac function

Once CO measurement is completed, other hemodynamic parameters can be calculated to complete the hemodynamic profile. Values needed to complete the hemodynamic profile include the patient's body surface area (BSA), mean arterial pressure (MAP), central venous (or right atrial) pressure, mean PA pressure (MPAP), and PA wedge or occlusion pressure (PAWP or PAOP).

To determine the patient's BSA, locate the patient's height in the left column of the nomogram (see the accompanying figure) and their weight in the right column, and use a ruler to draw a straight line connecting the two points. The point where the line intersects the BSA column indicates the patient's BSA in square meters.

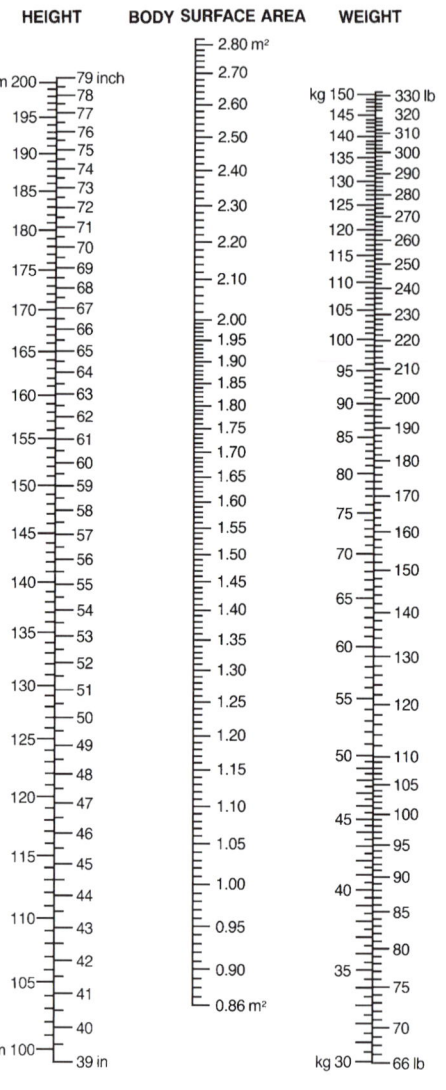

The nomogram shown here lets you plot the patient's height and weight to determine the BSA.

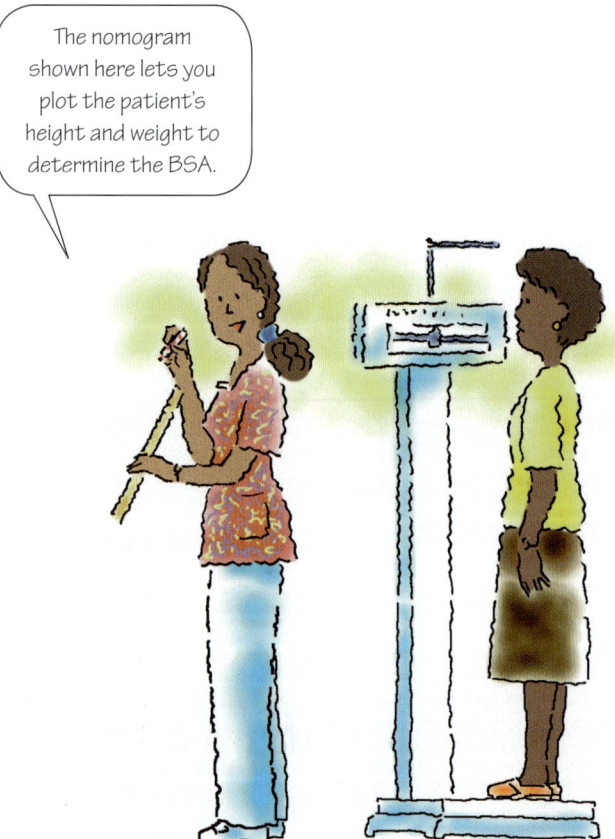

After you have completed the hemodynamic profile, calculate the cardiac index (CI), SV, stroke volume index (SVI), SVR, or pulmonary vascular resistance (PVR) using the formulas indicated in the following sections. For continuity, the same values for CO, HR, and SV will be used throughout the equations. Most monitoring systems compute these values automatically.

How to calculate the CI

The CI takes into account the patient's size when calculating cardiac flow. To calculate the CI, divide the CO value by the patient's BSA. Normally, the CI ranges from 2.5 to 4 L/min/m^2 (of BSA). For example, if a patient's CO is 5.5 L/min and their BSA is 1.64, CI would be 5.5/1.64, or 3.36 L/min/m^2.

How to calculate SV

To determine SV—the volume of blood pumped by the ventricle in one contraction—multiply the CO by 1,000 and divide by the HR. Normal SV ranges between 60 and 100 mL/beat.

$$SV = \frac{CO \times 1{,}000}{HR}$$

Example

Here, the patient's CO is 5.5 L/min and their HR is 80 beats/min.

$$SV = \frac{5.5 \times 1{,}000}{80}$$

$$SV = \frac{5{,}500}{80}$$

$$SV = 68.75 \text{ mL/beat}$$

How to calculate SVI

To assess whether the patient's SV is adequate for their body size, compute the SVI. Do so by dividing the SV by the patient's BSA or by dividing their CI $\times$ 1,000 by their HR. Normally, the SVI ranges between 35 and 75 mL/beat/m^2 of BSA.

Method 1:

$$SVI = \frac{SV}{BSA}$$

Method 2:

$$SVI = \frac{CI}{HR} \times 1,000$$

Example

As we determined in the earlier example, the patient's SV is 68.75 mL/beat. The patient's BSA is 1.64 m², and their CI is 3.35 L/min/m².

Calculating the SVI using method 1

$$SV = \frac{68.75}{1.64}$$

$$SVI = 42 \text{ mL/beat/m}^2$$

Calculating the SVI using method 2

$$SV = \frac{3.35}{80} \times 1,000$$

$$SVI = 42 \text{ mL/beat/m}^2$$

How to calculate SVR

To assess SVR—the degree of left ventricular resistance known as afterload—deduct the central venous pressure (CVP) from the MAP. Divide this value by the CO value. Then multiply by a rounded conversion factor of 80 to compute the value into units of force (dynes/sec/cm^{-5}). Normal SVR ranges from 900 to 1,400 dynes/sec/cm^{-5}.

$$SVR = \frac{MAP - CVP}{CO} \times 80$$

Example

Here, the patient's MAP is 93, and their CVP is 6; the patient's CO remains 5.5. Note that 80 is the conversion factor.

$$SVR = \frac{93 - 6}{5.5} \times 80$$

$$SVR = \frac{6,960}{5.5}$$

$$SVR = 1,265 \text{ dynes/sec/cm}^{-5}$$

Calculating PVR

To measure PVR—or right ventricular afterload—deduct the PAWP or PAOP from the MPAP. Then divide the product by the CO value. To compute the value into units of force (dynes/sec/cm^{-5}), multiply the result by 80. Normal PVR values range from 100 to 250 dynes/sec/cm^{-5}.

$$PVR = \frac{MPAP - PAWP}{CO} \times 80$$

Example

Here, the patient's MPAP is 20, and their PAWP or PAOP is 5; the patient's CO remains 5.5. Again, the conversion factor is 80.

$$PVR = \frac{20 - 5}{5.5} \times 80$$

$$PVR = \frac{1,200}{5.5}$$

$$PVR = 218 \text{ dynes/sec/cm}^{-5}$$

The nurse's role in CO monitoring

Nursing responsibilities

- Maintain PAC per institutional guidelines.
- Monitor right atrium and PA waveforms to verify proper catheter position.
- Measure and document CO and other hemodynamic parameters as prescribed or indicated.
- Include the fluid volume used for bolus CO measurement in the patient's intake and output.

- Change the system components (injectate tubing, solution, etc.) with the hemodynamic monitoring system (every 96 hours or per institutional policy).
- Correlate changes in hemodynamic measurements with patient assessment as well as changes in patient condition or medication administration.

> CO that falls below or above the mean can signal trouble. Use these strategies to avoid inaccurate measurements.

Troubleshooting

Use this chart to help you recognize and resolve common problems.

Problem	Causes	Nursing interventions
CO values lower than expected	Erroneous CC (set too low)	• Before injection, verify that the CC setting and the injectate volume are compatible.
	Injectate lumen exiting in right ventricle	• Confirm proper placement of the injectate lumen by observing the monitor for right atrial waveforms.
CO values higher than expected	Erroneous CC (set too high)	• Before injection, verify that the CC setting and the injectate volume are compatible. • Ensure an air-free system.
	Catheter tip too far into PA	• Check catheter placement by obtaining a PAWP/PAOP tracing. If the catheter is placed correctly, 1.25–1.5 mL of air will be necessary to obtain a PAWP/PAOP tracing. • Assist the provider to reposition the catheter, if necessary.
CO values deviating at least 10% from the mean (no pattern)	Arrhythmias, such as premature ventricular contractions and atrial fibrillation	• Observe the cardiac monitor while monitoring CO and instill injectate during a period without arrhythmias. • Increase the number of serial injections to five or six, and average the values. • If the arrhythmias continue, notify the provider.
	Catheter fling (turbulent, erratic waveform resulting from turbulence of blood circulating around intrusive catheter)	• Observe the waveforms and assist the provider in repositioning the catheter, if necessary. • If catheter fling does not decrease spontaneously after the catheter is inserted or repositioned, increase the number of serial CO determinations.
	Varying PA baseline temperature (which causes drift during respiration)	• Obtain CO values when respirations are steadier and less labored. • Instill injectate consistently at end-expiration. • Increase the number of serial injections.
	Variations in venous return (e.g., from rapid bolus administration of fluids or from the patient shivering or coughing)	• Avoid giving bolus injections of drugs or fluids just before measuring CO. • If shivering accompanies a fever, notify the provider. • Avoid measuring CO until coughing and restlessness subside.
	Inadequate signal-to-noise ratio	• To strengthen the signal, increase the injectate volume or lower the injectate temperature (e.g., by using iced injectate for patients with hypothermia).
	Poor injection technique	• Observe the upstroke on the thermodilution curve to detect an error in injection technique. • Use two hands to deliver a bolus injection quickly and evenly in less than 4 seconds.

Quick quiz

Color my world

Use a red pen or pencil to trace the path of injectate through the heart illustration.

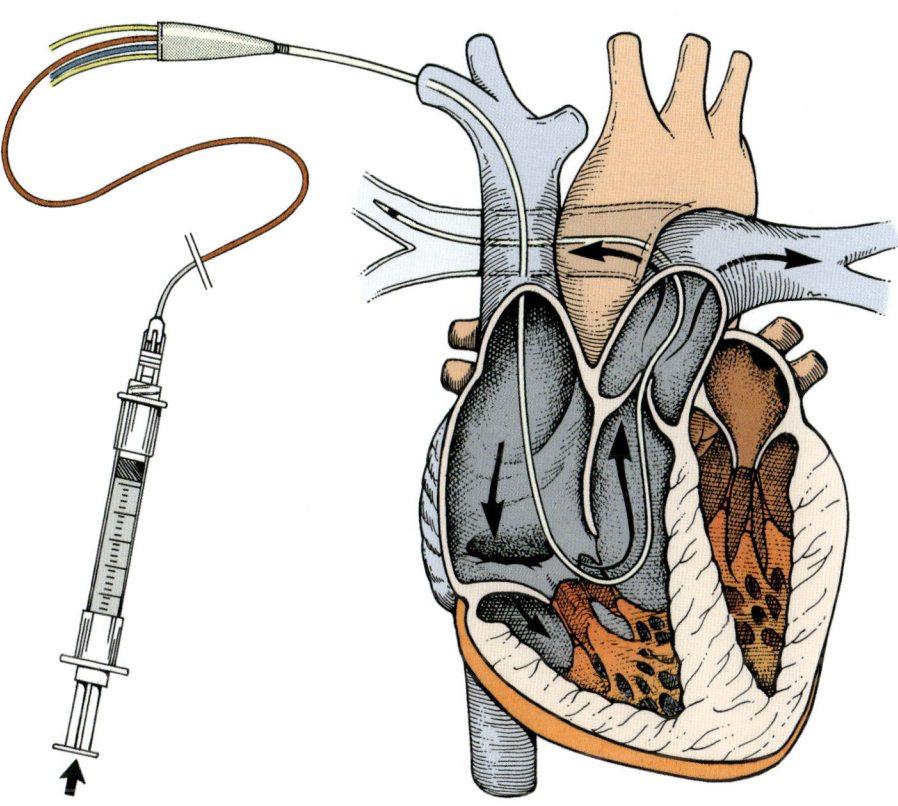

What do you know?

1. The most long-standing and reliable method of CO measurement is_____.

2. Indicate whether each of the below CO assessment methods is categorized as noninvasive, minimally invasive, or invasive.
    A. esophageal Doppler _____
    B. Fick method _____
    C. bioreactance _____
    D. arterial pulse wave analysis _____
    E. thermodilution _____

3. Which of the following statements is a technique used when measuring bolus thermodilution CO?
   A. inject volume over 15 seconds at end-inspiration
   B. ensure correct CC is utilized
   C. inject volume into the PA port
   D. ensure temperature difference of less than 10 degrees

Matchmaker

Match the following parameters with their descriptions.

1. Stroke volume _____

2. Systemic vascular resistance _____

3. Pulmonary vascular resistance _____

4. Cardiac index _____

A. Reflects left ventricular afterload

B. CO reflective of patient's height and weight

C. Volume of blood pumped by the ventricle in one contraction

D. Reflects right ventricular afterload

Answers: Color my world: The cold injectate is introduced into the right atrium through the proximal injection port. Then it flows into the right ventricle, where it mixes completely with the blood. Lastly, it flows into the PA; What do you know?: 1. thermodilution, 2A. minimally invasive, 2B. invasive, 2C. noninvasive, 2D. minimally invasive, 2E. invasive, 3. B; Matchmaker: 1. C, 2. A, 3. D, 4. B

Selected references

Delgado, S. (2023). *AACN essentials of critical care nursing* (5th ed.). McGraw-Hill.

Diepenbrock, N. (2020). *Quick reference to critical care* (6th ed.). Lippincott Williams & Wilkins.

Hartjes, T. (Ed.). (2022). *Core curriculum for high acuity, progressive and critical care nursing* (8th ed.). W.B. Saunders Co.

Johnson, K. (Ed.). (2023). *AACN procedure manual for progressive and critical care* (8th ed.). Elsevier.

Lippincott's nursing procedures & skills (10th ed.). (2022). Lippincott Williams & Wilkins.

McLaughlin, M. A. (2025). *Cardiovascular care made incredibly easy* (5th ed.). Wolters Kluwer.

Ruste, M., Jacquet-Lagreze, M., & Fellahi, J. L. (2023, June 1). Advantages and limitations of noninvasive devices for cardiac output monitoring: A literature review. *Current Opinion in Critical Care, 29*(3), 259–267. https://doi.org/10.1097/MCC.0000000000001045

Scheeren, T. W. L., & Ramsay, M. A. E. (2019). New developments in hemodynamic monitoring. *Journal of Cardiothoracic & Vascular Anesthesia, 33*(Suppl 1), S67–S72. https://doi.org/10.1053/j.jvca.2019.03.043

Singer, Z., Nagpal, D., Slessarev, M., Durocher, D., & Ward, M. R. (2023, April). The utility of invasive hemodynamics in the management of cardiogenic shock. *The Canadian Journal of Cardiology, 39*(4), 420–422. https://doi.org/10.1016/j.cjca.2023.02.002

Chapter 8

Tissue oxygenation monitoring

Understanding oxygen supply and tissue demand

Most oxygen (O_2) collected in the lungs binds with hemoglobin (Hb) to form oxyhemoglobin. However, a small portion of it dissolves in the plasma. The portion of oxygen that dissolves in the plasma can be measured as the partial pressure of arterial oxygen in the blood (PaO_2).

After oxygen binds to Hb, red blood cells (RBCs) carry it by way of the circulatory system to tissues throughout the body. Internal respiration occurs by cellular diffusion when RBCs release oxygen and absorb the carbon dioxide (CO_2) produced by cellular metabolism. The RBCs then transport the carbon dioxide back to the lungs for removal during expiration.

Most of the oxygen I collect binds with hemoglobin to form oxyhemoglobin.

Oxygen transport

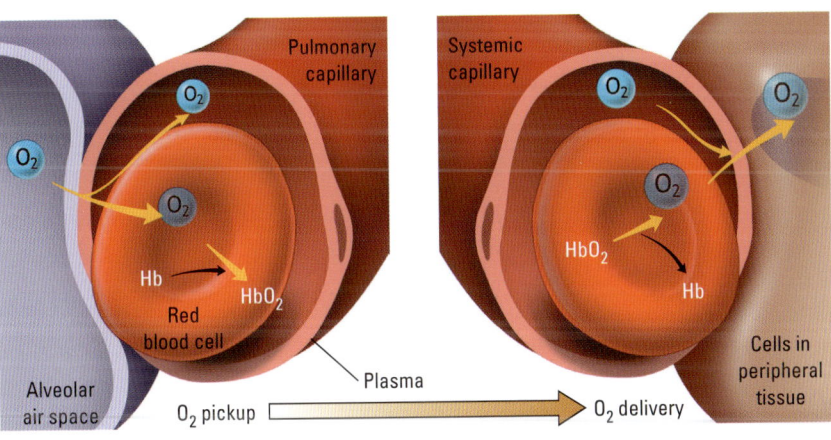

Pulmonary capillary

Systemic capillary

O_2

O_2

O_2

O_2

O_2

O_2

O_2

Hb

HbO_2

HbO_2

Hb

Red blood cell

Alveolar air space

Plasma

Cells in peripheral tissue

O_2 pickup

O_2 delivery

Carbon dioxide transport

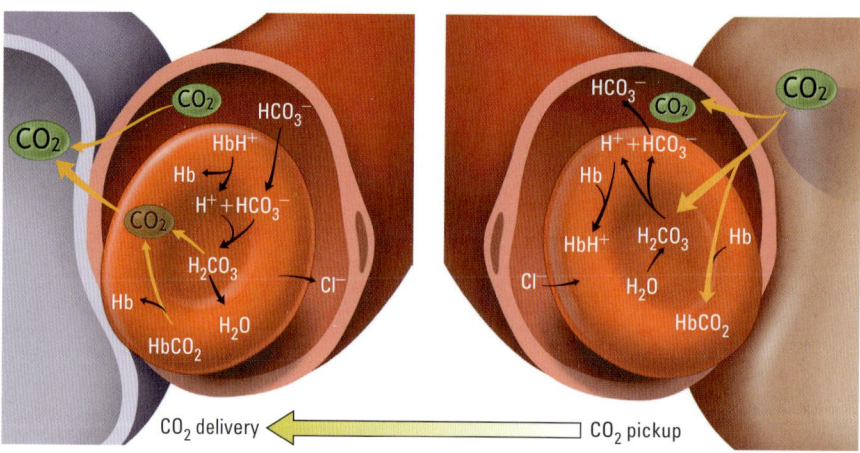

CO$_2$ delivery ⟵ CO$_2$ pickup

Venous oxygen reserve, arterial oxygen delivery, and oxygen consumption

The below figure illustrates the relationship between venous oxygen reserve, arterial oxygen delivery, and oxygen consumption. See the next page for explanations of these terms.

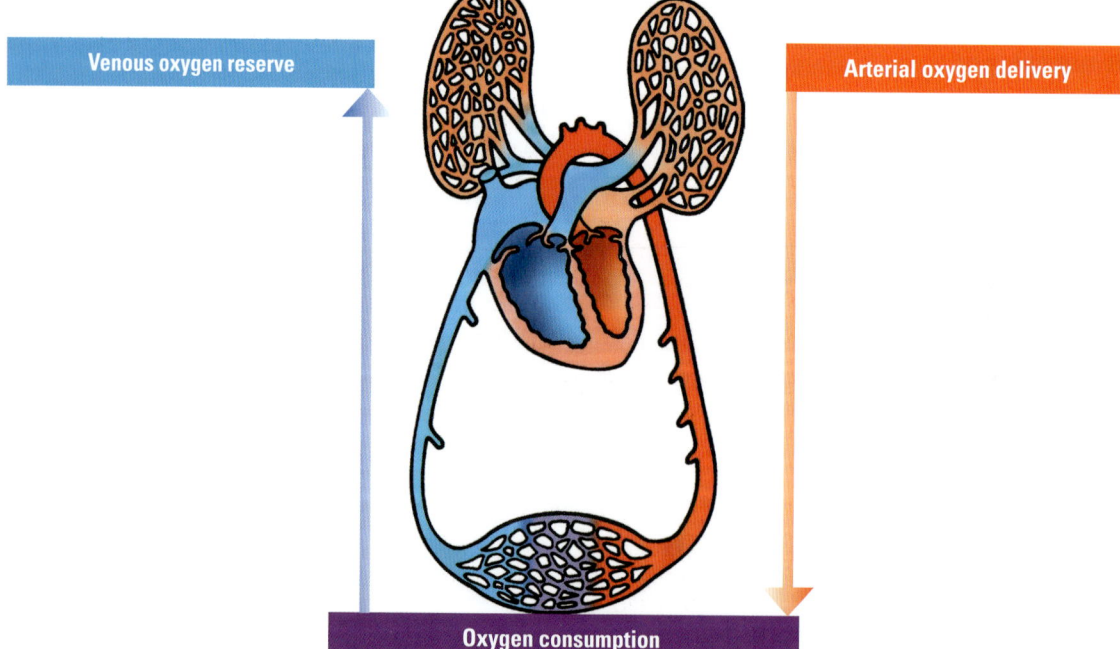

Venous oxygen reserve

Venous oxygen reserve (Rvo$_2$) is the amount of oxygen left over (not used by body tissues) that returns to the heart in venous blood. Rvo$_2$ depends on two factors:
- arterial oxygen delivery (Dao$_2$)
- oxygen consumption.
  Normal Rvo$_2$ ranges from 700 to 800 mL O$_2$/min, or 450 mL O$_2$/min/m^2 based on body surface area (BSA).

Arterial oxygen delivery

The amount of oxygen transported to the tissues, Dao$_2$, depends on two factors:
- arterial oxygen content—the total amount of oxygen in the blood that's available to tissue cells
- cardiac output (CO)—the amount of blood pumped out of the heart per minute.
  Normal Dao$_2$ ranges from 900 to 1,000 mL O$_2$/min, or 600 mL O$_2$/min/m^2 based on BSA.

Oxygen consumption

The amount of oxygen used by the tissues in the body is called oxygen consumption. Oxygen consumption is determined by three factors:
- oxygen demand (the cells' requirement for oxygen)
- oxygen delivery (the supply of oxygen delivered to the tissues)
- transport of oxygen from the blood for use by the cells.
  Normal oxygen consumption ranges from 200 to 240 mL O$_2$/min, or 150 mL O$_2$/min/m^2 based on BSA.

A closer look at Sao$_2$

Arterial oxygen saturation (Sao$_2$), expressed as a percentage, represents the actual amount of oxygen bound to Hb divided by the maximum amount of oxygen that could possibly bind to Hb. Because Hb carries most of the blood's oxygen, a normal Sao$_2$ level is 95% to 100%. Pulse oximetry is a noninvasive, real-time estimation of the oxygen saturation of Hb in arterial blood.

Factors affecting Sao$_2$

Certain conditions impair the body's oxygen supply system, resulting in decreased Sao$_2$, thereby threatening adequate tissue oxygenation. These conditions include those that cause:
- decreased CO, such as heart failure and shock.
- inadequate binding of oxygen to Hb, such as carbon monoxide poisoning, nitrate or nitrite therapy, certain anesthetics, and sulfonamide therapy.

- severe anemia (inadequate amounts of Hb).
- increased tissue oxygen requirements, such as thyroid storm, malignant hyperthermia, extremely prolonged exercise, delirium tremens, and status epilepticus.
- inability of tissue cells to absorb or use the oxygen they receive, such as sepsis, cyanide toxicity, and ethanol toxicity.

How the body responds to decreased Sa_{O_2}

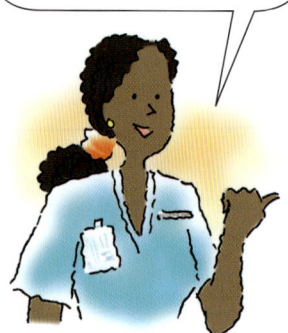

To maintain normal tissue oxygenation and avoid hypoxia, the body needs to compensate for these conditions. Let's see what can happen…

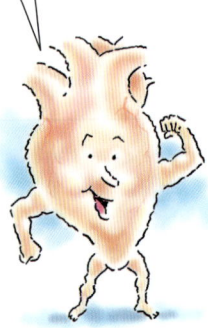

I increase my output to quickly deliver more blood to body tissues!

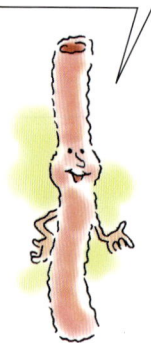

An increased extraction of oxygen from systemic capillaries helps out!

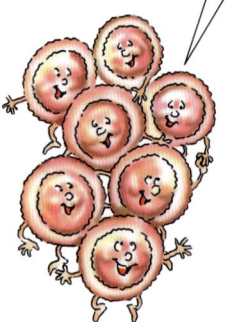

An increased amount of hemoglobin can help, too. However, it might be too slow a process to benefit those who are acutely ill.

How pulse oximetry works

Performed intermittently or continuously, oximetry is a simple procedure used to monitor arterial oxygen saturation noninvasively. Pulse oximeters usually indicate arterial oxygen saturation values with the symbol Sp_{O_2}, whereas invasively measured arterial oxygen saturation values are indicated by the symbol Sa_{O_2}.

This distinction is important given the differences in the methods of the readings. The Sa_{O_2} is much more precise because it is a directly measured value as opposed to the real-time estimation of the Sp_{O_2}.

In pulse oximetry, two light-emitting diodes (LEDs) send red and infrared light through a pulsating arterial vascular bed such as the one in the fingertip or the earlobe. A photodetector slipped over the finger or earlobe measures the transmitted light as it passes through the vascular bed, detects the relative amount of color absorbed by arterial blood, and provides an estimated arterial oxygen saturation.

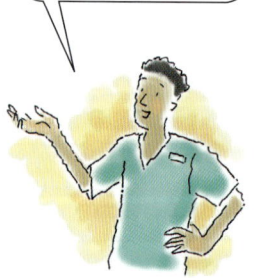

No bones about it. Pulse oximetry can provide an accurate estimate of arterial oxygen saturation without interference from venous blood, skin, tissue—or even bone!

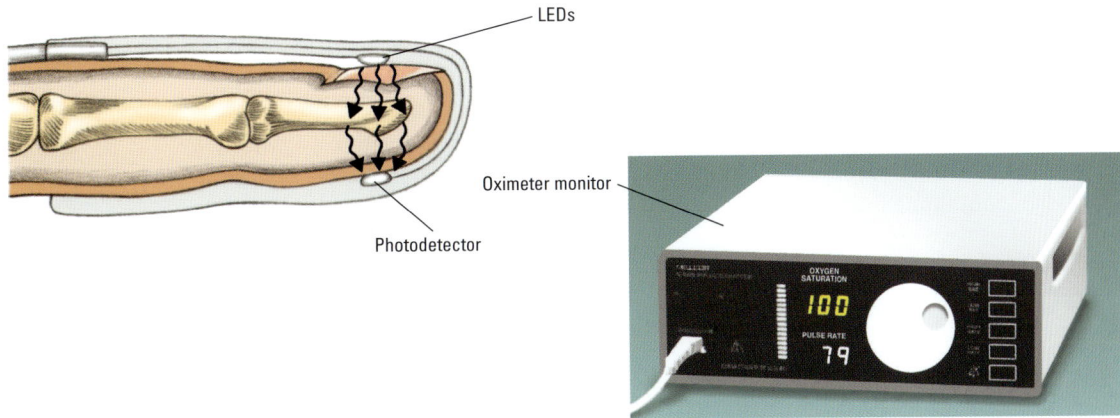

LEDs

Oximeter monitor

Photodetector

OXYGEN
SATURATION

100

PULSE RATE

79

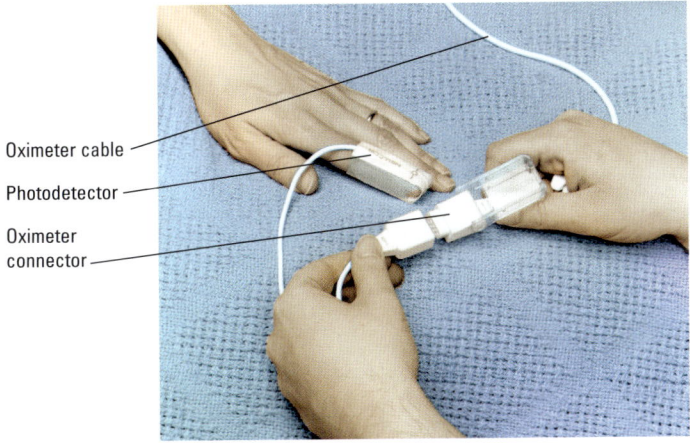

Oximeter cable

Photodetector

Oximeter
connector

How to use pulse oximetry

Finger probe

1. Select one finger for the test. Although the index finger is commonly used, a smaller finger may be selected if the patient's fingers are too large for the equipment. Make sure the patient isn't wearing false fingernails, and remove nail polish from the test finger. Place the transducer (photodetector) probe over the patient's finger so that light beams and sensors oppose each other. If the patient has long fingernails, position the probe perpendicular to the finger, if possible, or clip the fingernail. Always position the patient's hand at heart level to eliminate venous pulsations and to promote accurate readings.
2. If you're testing a neonate or a small infant, wrap the probe around the foot so that light beams and detectors oppose each other. For a large infant, use a probe that fits on the great toe and secure it to the foot.

3. Turn on the power switch. If the device is working properly, a beep will sound, a display will light momentarily, and the pulse searchlight will flash. The SpO_2 (indicating arterial oxygen saturation by pulse oximetry) and pulse rate displays will show stationary zeros. After four to six heartbeats, the SpO_2 and pulse rate display will supply information with each beat, and the pulse amplitude indicator will begin tracking the pulse.

Ear probe

1. Following the manufacturer's instructions, attach the ear probe to the patient's earlobe or pinna. Use the ear probe stabilizer for prolonged or exercise testing. Be sure to establish good contact on the ear; an unstable probe may set off the low-perfusion alarm. After the probe has been attached for a few seconds, a saturation reading and pulse waveform will appear on the oximeter's screen.

2. After the procedure, remove the ear probe, turn off and unplug the unit, and clean the probe by gently rubbing it with an alcohol pad.

3. Leave the ear probe in place for 3 or more minutes until readings stabilize at the highest point, or take three separate readings and average them.

Troubleshooting the pulse oximetry system

When using pulse oximetry to measure arterial oxygen saturation, there are several problems that can be avoided or fixed by following good clinical practice.

Avoiding pulse oximetry interference

Certain factors can interfere with the accuracy of oximetry readings:

- Elevated bilirubin levels (which may falsely lower oxygen saturation readings) or carboxyhemoglobin or methemoglobin levels (which may falsely elevate oxygen saturation readings)
- Intravascular substances, such as lipid emulsions and dyes
- Excessive light (such as from phototherapy or direct sunlight), patient movement, or ear pigment
- Hypothermia
- Hypotension
- Vasoconstriction
- Some acrylic nails and certain colors of nail polish (blue, green, black, and brown-red).

Best practices when using pulse oximetry

- To maintain a continuous display of arterial oxygen saturation levels, the monitoring site must be clean and dry.
- If the skin becomes irritated from adhesives used to keep disposable probes in place, change the oximetry site. You can also

replace disposable probes that irritate the skin with nondisposable models.

- Obtaining a signal can be a problem with pulse oximeters. If you encounter this issue, first check the patient's vital signs. If they're sufficient enough to produce a signal, use the chart below to check for problems and intervene.

Troubleshooting tips

Problem	Interventions
Poor connection	• Check that the sensors are aligned properly. • Make sure that the wires are intact and fastened securely and that the pulse oximeter is plugged into a power source.
Inadequate or intermittent blood flow to the site	• Check the patient's pulse rate and capillary refill time, and take corrective action if blood flow to the site is decreased. Such action may include loosening restraints, removing tight-fitting clothes, taking off a blood pressure cuff, or checking arterial and IV lines. • If none of these interventions work, find an alternative site. Finding a site with proper circulation may also prove challenging when a patient is receiving vasoconstrictive drugs.
Equipment malfunctions	• Remove the pulse oximeter from the patient, set the alarm limits according to your facility's policies, and try the instrument on yourself or another healthy person. Doing so will tell you whether the equipment is working correctly.

A closer look at Sv̄o₂

After oxygen is delivered to the tissues, some remains attached to Hb and returns to the heart in venous blood. Mixed venous oxygen saturation (Sv̄o₂) is the oxygen saturation of Hb in venous blood that returns to the heart from the tissues. Normal Sv̄o₂ levels are also expressed in percentages, ranging from 60% to 80%. Sv̄o₂ levels are determined by tissue oxygen consumption and CO (the amount of blood pumped out of the heart per minute).

Arterial blood with oxygen-saturated Hb (normally 96% to 100% saturated) is delivered to body tissues, where cells extract and use about 25% of this oxygen. Then, the blood passes into venous circulation, now with Hb only 60% to 80% saturated with oxygen because the cells have taken about 25%. This venous blood is returned to the heart, where Sv̄o₂ measurements are made in the pulmonary artery (PA).

An alternative to measuring Sv̄o₂ in the PA is central venous monitoring of oxygen saturation Sv̄o₂, where a catheter is placed in the superior vena cava or upper right atrium. The location of the catheter tip is important for accuracy to allow the measurement from the junction of the superior vena cava-right atrium.

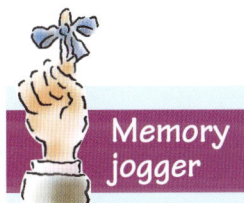

Memory jogger

Arterial blood with oxygen-saturated hemoglobin (normally 96% to 100% saturated) is delivered to body tissues, where cells extract and use about 25% of this oxygen. To remember this, think of it visually—that is, **picture about one quarter of the oxygen-saturated hemoglobin being used.**

In addition, tissue oxygenation saturation (StO_2), the ratio of oxygenated hemoglobin to total hemoglobin in the microcirculation, can be measured through a noninvasive method. It also assesses the amount of oxygen extraction.

Factors affecting $S\bar{v}O_2$

The patient's $S\bar{v}O_2$ level alone isn't useful information. The balance between available oxygen and tissue consumption depends on other factors, such as CO, SaO_2, and Hb levels on the supply side and tissue oxygen needs on the demand side. Any change in the patient's $S\bar{v}O_2$ level typically reflects a change in one or more of these factors.

Increased $S\bar{v}O_2$

Conditions that raise $S\bar{v}O_2$ levels and lower the demand for oxygen include:

- anesthesia
- chemical paralysis
- elevated SaO_2 levels
- hypothermia
- increased CO
- increased Hb level
- sedation
- shunting in the microcirculation.

Decreased $S\bar{v}O_2$

Conditions that lower $S\bar{v}O_2$ levels and raise the demand for oxygen include:

- cardiogenic shock
- decreased CO
- decreased Hb level
- hyperthermia or fever
- reduced SaO_2 levels
- seizures
- septic shock
- shivering.

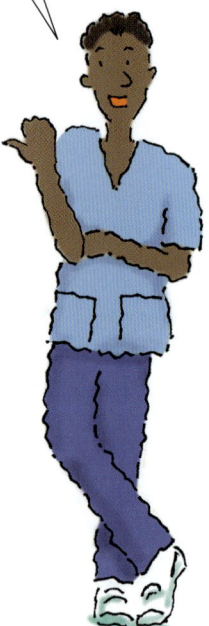

Increased CO can increase $S\bar{v}O_2$ levels.

$S\bar{v}O_2$ monitoring

$S\bar{v}O_2$ monitoring uses a fiberoptic thermodilution PA catheter to continuously monitor oxygen delivery to tissues and oxygen consumption by tissues. Monitoring of $S\bar{v}O_2$ allows rapid detection of impaired oxygen delivery, as from decreased CO, Hb level, or SaO_2. It also helps evaluate a patient's response to drug therapy, endotracheal tube suctioning, ventilator setting changes, positive end-expiratory pressure, and fraction of inspired oxygen. Ongoing monitoring allows trending, which may be more meaningful than a single reading.

Central venous oxygen saturation ($S\bar{v}o_2$) monitoring requires the placement of a central venous catheter with additional fiberoptics and a specialized monitor to continuously monitor venous oxygen saturation.

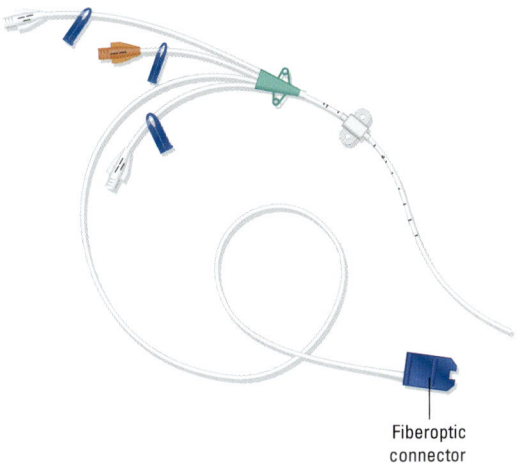

Fiberoptic
connector

Sto₂ monitoring

Noninvasive tissue oxygen saturation (Sto_2) monitoring can assist in the early detection of inadequate regional tissue perfusion. It requires a disposable sensor that's placed on the thenar eminence of the hand and a specialized monitor. Near-infrared light illuminates the muscle tissue; the returned light produces a measurement of oxygen saturation in the microcirculation.

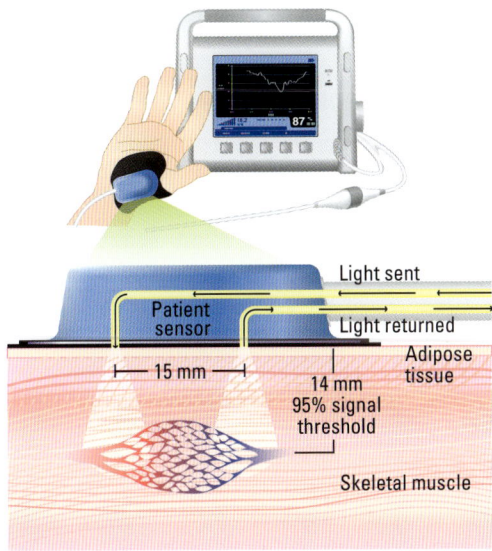

Light sent

Patient
sensor

Light returned

Adipose
tissue

15 mm

14 mm
95% signal
threshold

Skeletal muscle

Troubleshooting the system

If the intensity of the tracing is low:
- ensure that all connections between the catheter and oximeter are secure.
- ensure that the catheter is patent and not kinked.
  If the tracing is damped or erratic:
- try to aspirate blood from the catheter to check for patency (if allowed by your facility).

If you can't aspirate blood:
- notify the provider so that the catheter can be replaced.
- check the PA waveform to determine whether the catheter has wedged.

If the catheter has wedged:
- turn the patient from side to side and instruct to cough.

If the catheter remains wedged:
- notify the provider immediately.

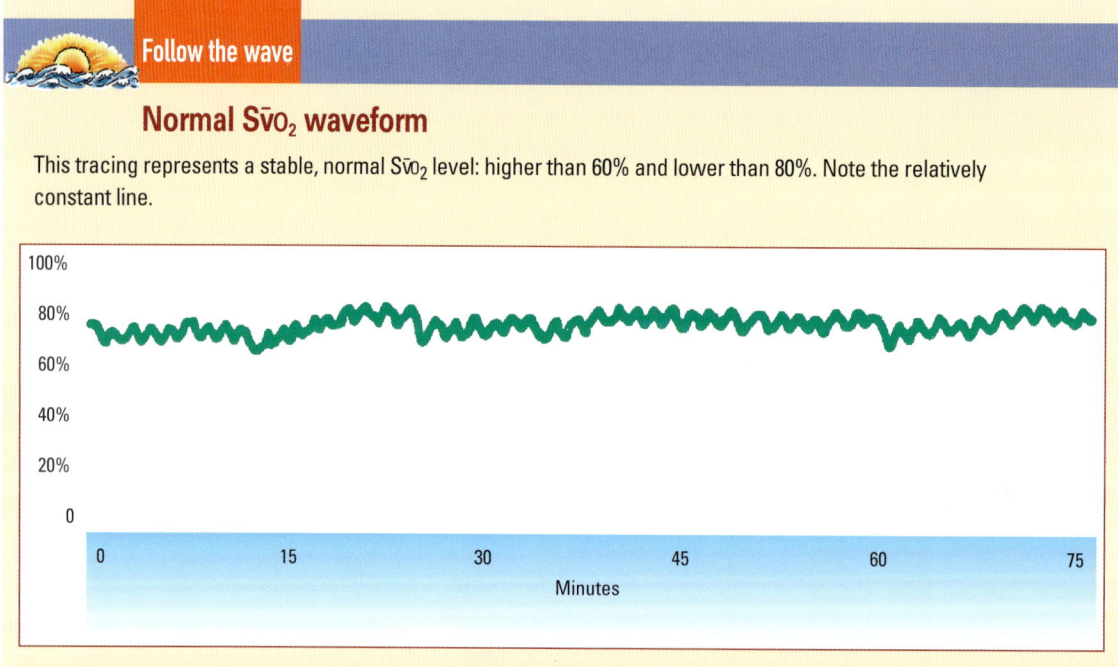

Follow the wave

Normal S$\bar{v}o_2$ waveform

This tracing represents a stable, normal S$\bar{v}o_2$ level: higher than 60% and lower than 80%. Note the relatively constant line.

Follow the wave

Abnormal Sv̄o₂ waveforms

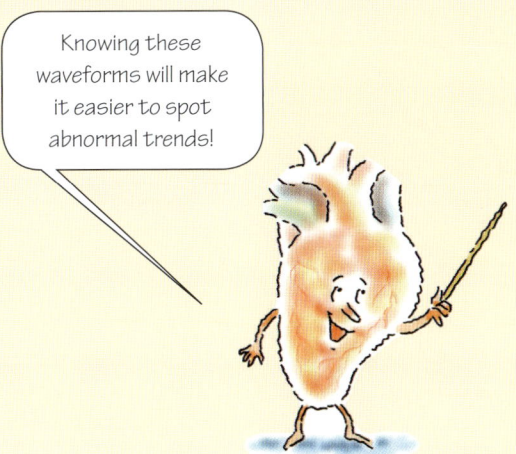

Knowing these waveforms will make it easier to spot abnormal trends!

The first tracing shows a falling venous oxygen saturation (Sv̄o₂) level in a patient returning from the operating room after coronary artery bypass surgery. Notice the event marks that indicate atrial pacing and the cardiac index (CI) at about 1 hour, 15 minutes; administration of a vasoactive drug; the patient's plotted response; and the patient's subsequent return to the operating room.

Because a patient's Sv̄o₂ level may change almost immediately after intervention, the subsequent levels can help you determine the intervention's effectiveness. This tracing shows a rise in Sv̄o₂ levels and CO after the patient has received IV nitroprusside.

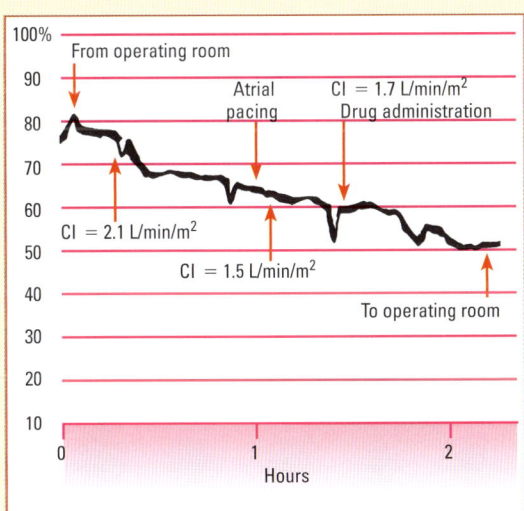

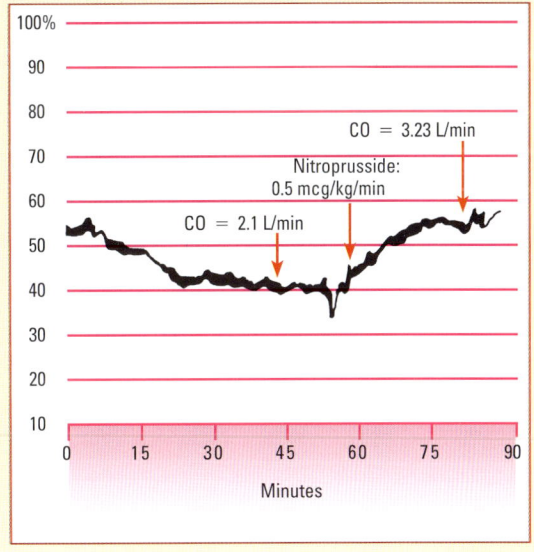

This tracing represents the patient's response to a muscle relaxant.

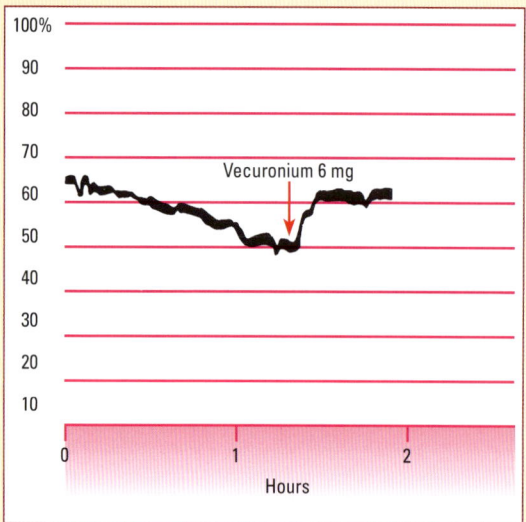

This waveform shows the patient's response to changes in ventilator settings. Note that increasing the positive end-expiratory pressure (PEEP) causes an increase in $S\bar{v}o_2$; therefore, the fraction of inspired oxygen (Fio_2) can be decreased.

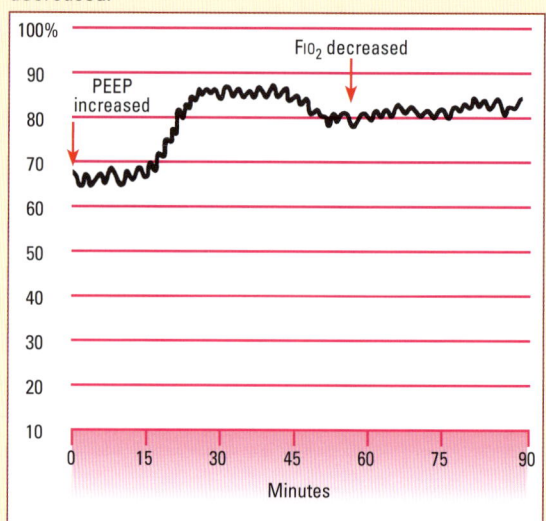

This waveform shows typical changes in the $S\bar{v}o_2$ level as a result of various activities.

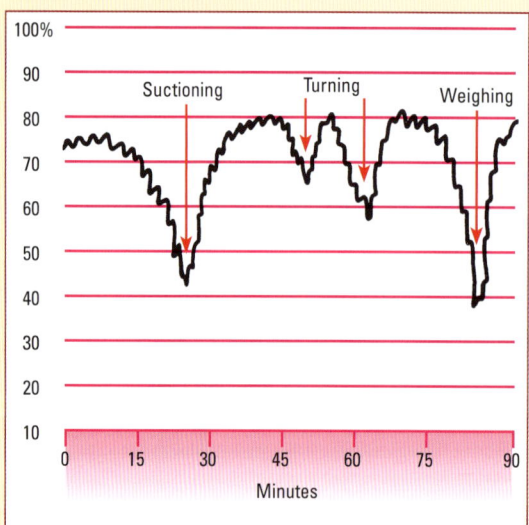

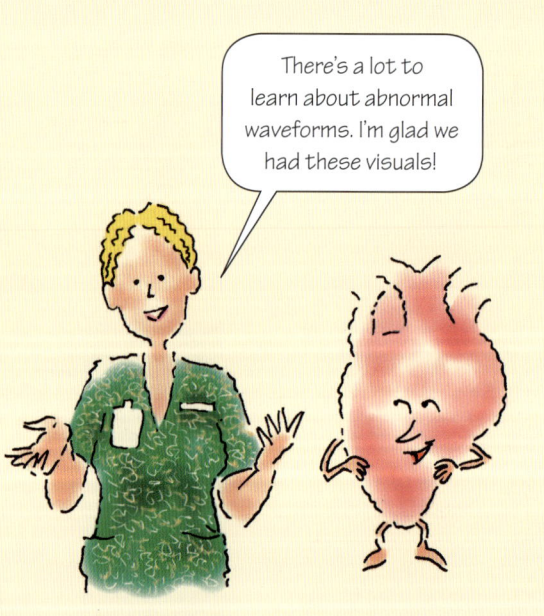

There's a lot to learn about abnormal waveforms. I'm glad we had these visuals!

Recent advances

During the last few decades, the importance of the microcirculation has been recognized in relation to managing and optimizing optimal tissue oxygenation. The development of new technologies that are able to measure and evaluate the microcirculation has provided a greater insight into managing hemodynamic stability much more precisely. Clinical research has shed light on the importance of an overall "big-picture" evaluation of tissue oxygenation optimization rather than on spot checks using general measurement techniques. Methods such as plethysmography and total hemoglobin concentration (SpHb) continue to offer opportunities to refine technology to better manage patients.

Quick quiz

Show and tell

Identify the type or cause of the $S\bar{v}O_2$ waveform shown in each of these illustrations.

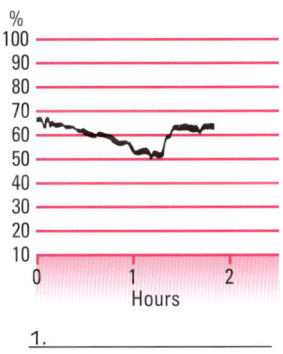

1. _____

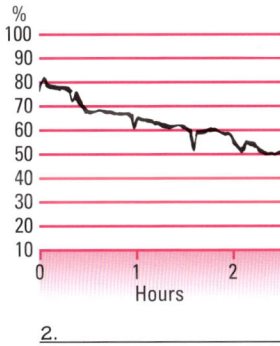

2. _____

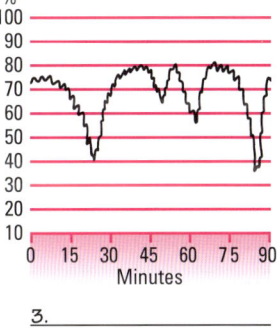

3. _____

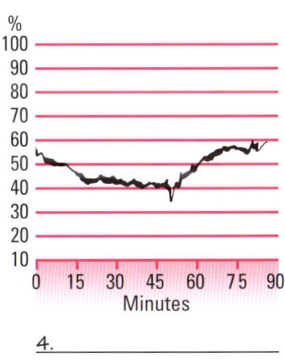

4. _____

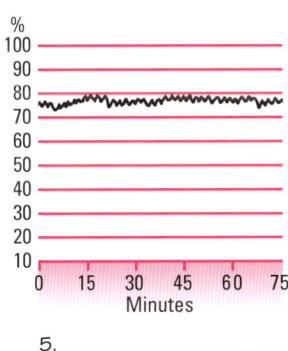

5. _____

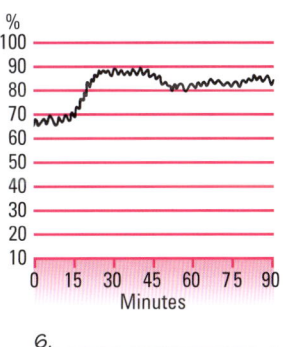

6. _____

Matchmaker

Match each abbreviation with the correct spelled-out version of the term.

1. DaO_2 _____   A. partial pressure of arterial oxygen

2. SaO_2 _____   B. arterial oxygen delivery

3. $S\bar{v}O_2$ _____   C. venous oxygen reserve

4. PaO_2 _____   D. arterial oxygen saturation

5. RvO_2 _____   E. mixed venous oxygen saturation

Answers: Show and tell: 1. Patient response to a muscle relaxant, 2. Falling $S\bar{v}O_2$ level, 3. Typical changes in the $S\bar{v}O_2$ level as a result of various activities (suctioning, turning, weighing), 4. Rise in $S\bar{v}O_2$ levels and cardiac output, 5. Normal $S\bar{v}O_2$ waveform, 6. Patient response to change in ventilator settings; Matchmaker: 1. B, 2. D, 3. E, 4. A, 5. C

Selected references

American Thoracic Society. (2019). *Pulse oximetry—American Thoracic Society Education Series*. American Thoracic Society Patient Education Series. https://www .thoracic.org/patients/patient-resources/resources/pulse-oximetry.pdf

Massari, D., Sahinovic, M., Flick, M., Vos, J. J., & Scheeren, T. W. (2022). What is new in microcirculation and tissue oxygenation monitoring? *Journal of Clinical Monitoring and Computing, 36*(2), 291–299. https://doi.org/10.1007/s10877-022-00837-x

Xu, L., Wang, M., Gong, S., Ye, C., & Wu, L. (2020). Transcutaneous oxygen pressure-related variables as noninvasive indicators of low lactate clearance in sepsis patients after resuscitation. *Journal of Clinical Monitoring and Computing, 35*(3), 435–442. https://doi.org/10.1007/s10877-020-00594-9

Xu, Z., Dong, P., & Zhou, X. (2023). Variation in central venous oxygen saturation to evaluate fluid responsiveness: A systematic review and meta-analysis. *Critical Care, 27*(1), 203. https://doi.org/10.1186/s13054-023-04480-z

Zorgati, A., Ben Soltane, H., & Nouira, S. (2021). Variation in central venous oxygen saturation to assess volume responsiveness in hemodynamically unstable patients under mechanical ventilation: A prospective cohort study. *Critical Care, 25*(1), 245. https://doi.org/10.1186/s13054-021-03683-6

Chapter 9

Minimally invasive and noninvasive hemodynamic monitoring

Although invasive hemodynamic monitoring using a pulmonary artery (PA) catheter remains the gold standard for clinical practice, minimally invasive monitoring techniques are proving to be reliable and safe options that yield results that relate with PA catheter readings.

Minimally invasive hemodynamic monitoring techniques are easier to use, can be applied in many clinical settings, and provide reproducible results.

Recent advances in technology to detect pulmonary pressures remotely from home help clinicians to manage the patient's volume status and to adjust diuretics. This is achieved by placement of a sensor, either through a right heart catheterization or noninvasively transdermally. Data support that remote monitoring of the patient's PA pressures allows a more proactive approach to fluid management. This technology detects the first change in the body that occurs in heart failure several days prior to the patient developing signs of shortness of breath or fluid on the body.

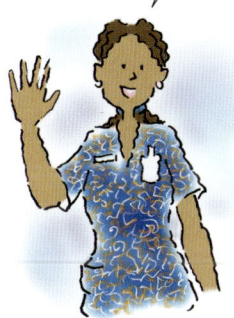

Transesophageal Doppler hemodynamic monitoring can keep track of five hemodynamic values—not bad for a minimally invasive monitoring system!

Transesophageal Doppler hemodynamic monitoring

Transesophageal Doppler hemodynamic monitoring is a minimally invasive method of using ultrasound to measure heart function. It involves placement of a probe into the esophagus. By measuring blood flow through the heart valves or ventricular outflow tracts, this monitoring system can monitor:

- cardiac output (CO)
- stroke volume (SV)
- cardiac index (CI)
- systemic vascular resistance (SVR)
- systemic vascular resistance index (SVRI).

Indications and contraindications for transesophageal Doppler hemodynamic monitoring

Indications

This type of monitoring is appropriate for:
- sedated, critically ill patients with difficult fluid management
- use during and after cardiac surgery
- patients undergoing major or high-risk surgery or high-risk patients undergoing any surgery excluding head, neck, and esophageal surgery
- patients treated in critical care requiring CO monitoring for any reason.

Contraindications

It is not recommended for patients:
- undergoing intra-aortic balloon pump (IABP) counterpulsation
- with severe coarctation of the aorta
- with a disorder of the pharynx, esophagus, or stomach
- with carcinoma of the esophagus or pharynx or previous esophageal surgery, esophageal stricture, varices, or pharyngeal pouch
- with a bleeding disorder
- with severe coagulopathies.

Pros and cons

Pros

- It is minimally invasive.
- Easier to insert, with rare complications

Cons

- It is difficult to align the ultrasound beam with the flow of blood. (If the beam is not properly angled, the results are not reliable.)
- It carries the risk of esophageal damage or perforation.
- The patient may require sedation because of the stiffness of the probe.

Transducer probe placement

Transducer probe placement for transesophageal Doppler hemodynamic monitoring is similar to inserting a nasogastric or orogastric tube, and it typically can be performed by a nurse at the bedside. However, the patient usually requires sedation for this procedure because the probe is rigid.

The nurse can typically perform the insertion of a transducer probe. However, the patient usually requires sedation.

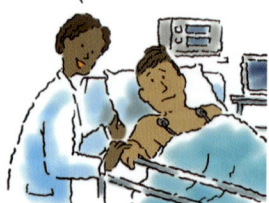

The stiff probe is lubricated and then inserted nasally or orally to a depth of 14 to 16 in (35.5 to 40.5 cm). Each probe has depth markers to demonstrate appropriate depth placement. The probe can be taped in place or left unsecured to allow for adjustments (if the patient is sedated). When the probe is positioned properly, it is ready to measure blood flow in the descending thoracic aorta.

First, the transducer probe is lubricated. It can then be inserted nasally or orally. Oral placement is shown here.

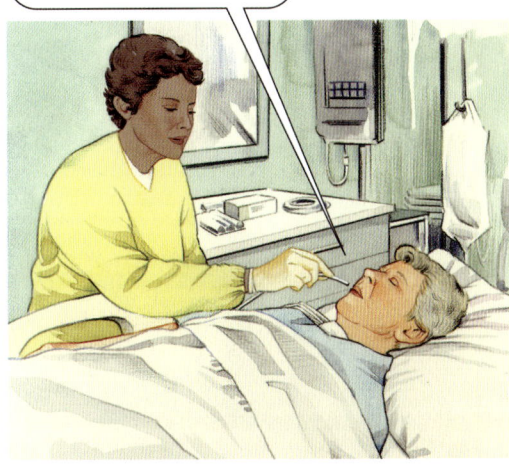

Depth markers on the probe enable easy insertion to a depth of 35.5 to 40.5 cm.

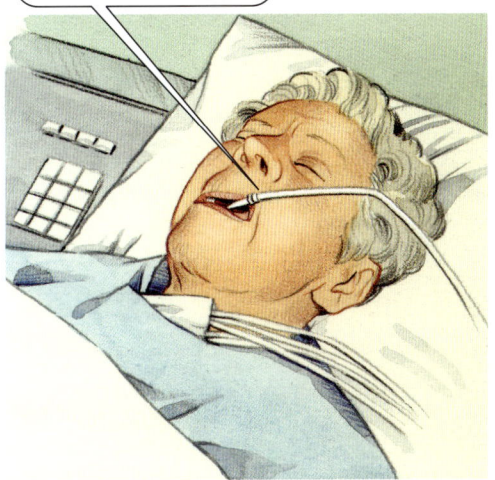

The probe can then be secured with tape or left unsecured (if the patient is sedated).

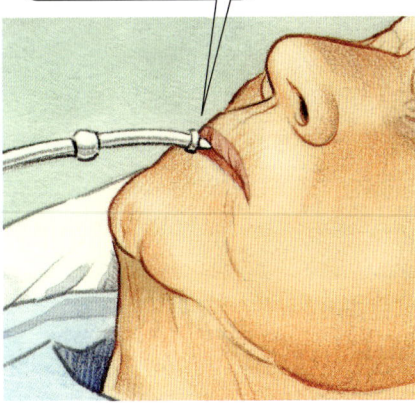

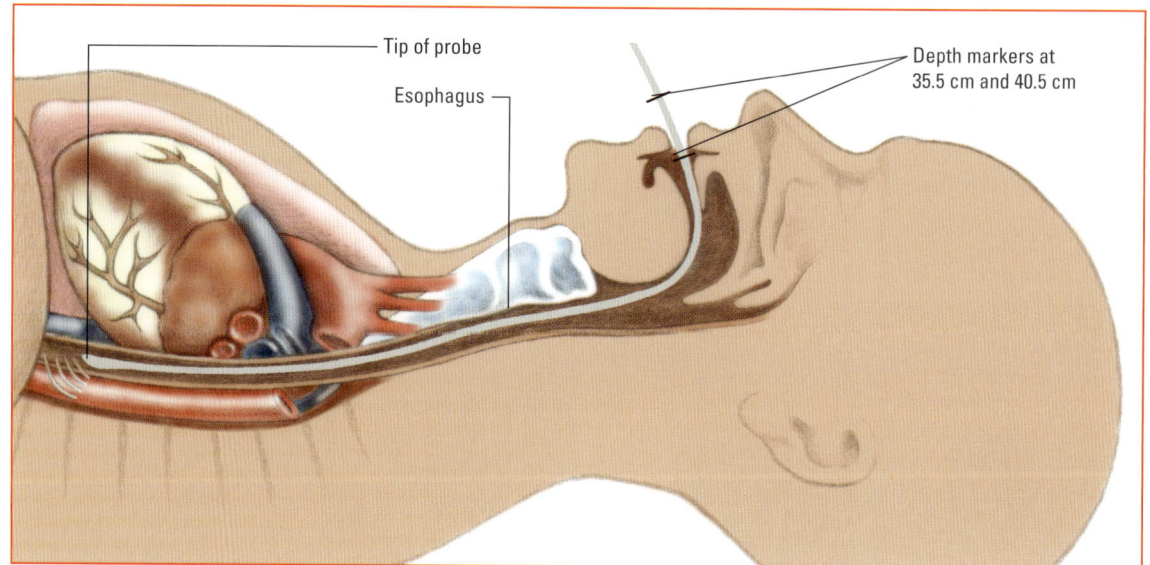

Tip of probe

Esophagus

Depth markers at 35.5 cm and 40.5 cm

Follow the wave

Transesophageal Doppler hemodynamic monitoring waveform

This normal waveform shows good capture of blood flow. Key aspects of the waveform include peak velocity (PV) and systolic blood flow in milliseconds or seconds, corrected for heart rate (HR).

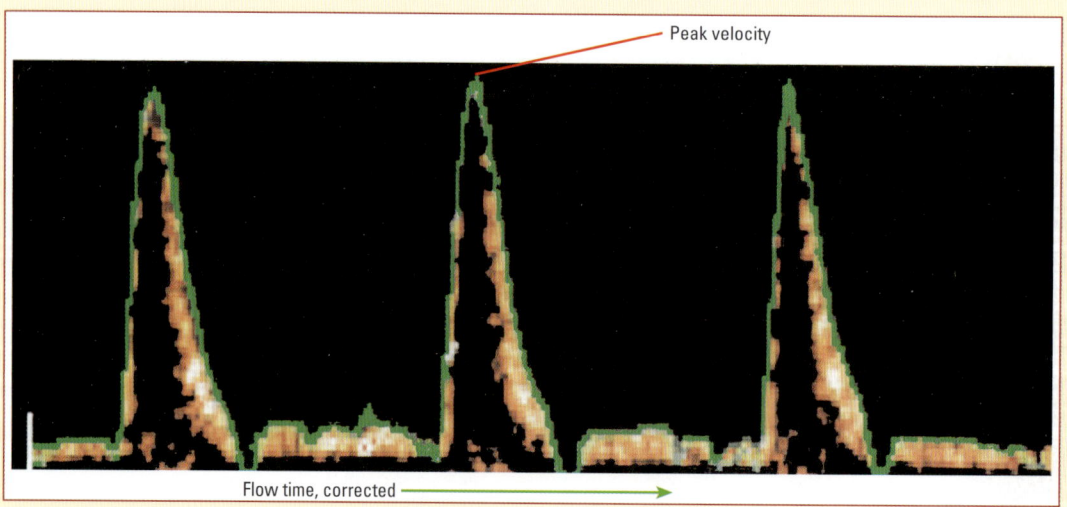

Peak velocity

Flow time, corrected

On the level

Normal values in esophageal Doppler hemodynamic monitoring

Parameter	Normal values
Flow time, corrected (the time in milliseconds or seconds of systolic blood flow, corrected to HR)	330–360 ms
PV (the velocity of the blood measured at the peak of systole)	20 years: 90–120 cm/sec 50 years: 60–90 cm/sec 70 years: 50–80 cm/sec

A closer look at the transesophageal Doppler hemodynamic monitoring system

This monitor automatically measures such values as HR, PV, flow time corrected (FTc), and more. Other hemodynamic monitoring parameters are then derived from these direct measurements, including CO, CI, SV, stroke volume index, and SVR.

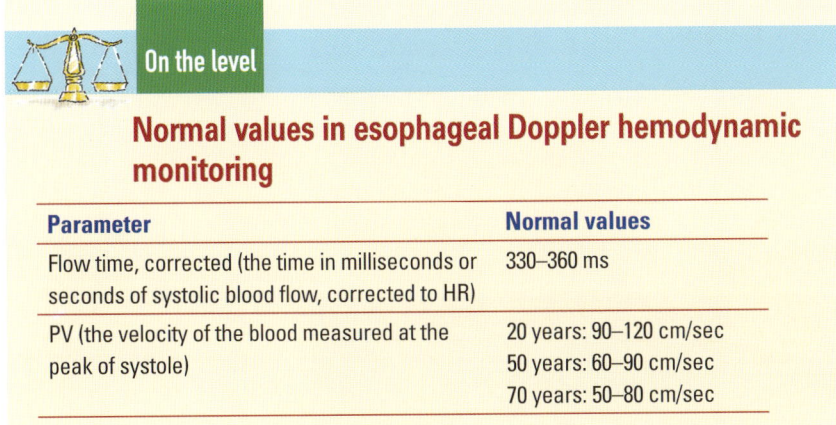

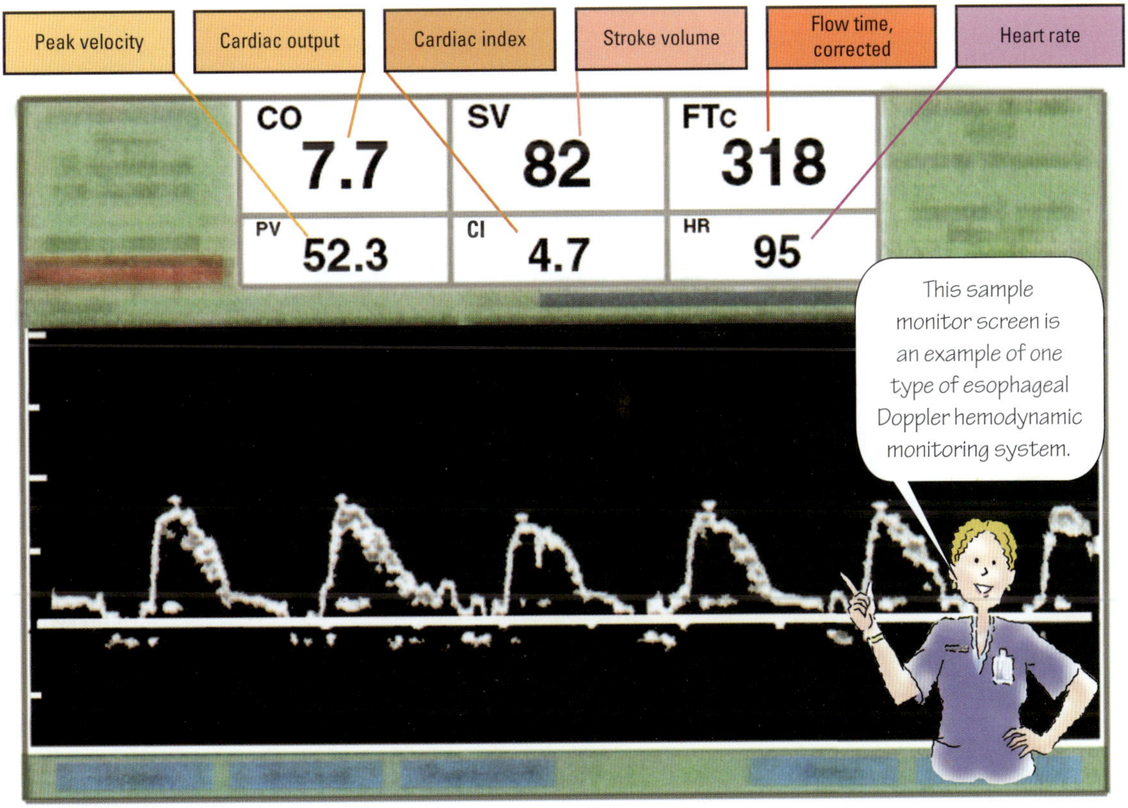

Peak velocity   Cardiac output   Cardiac index   Stroke volume   Flow time, corrected   Heart rate

CO	SV	FTc
7.7	82	318

PV	CI	HR
52.3	4.7	95

This sample monitor screen is an example of one type of esophageal Doppler hemodynamic monitoring system.

Arterial pressure—based CO monitoring

Arterial pressure–based cardiac output (APCO) monitoring provides a minimally invasive method to measure CO, which is SV multiplied by the patient's HR. In APCO monitoring, pulse pressure (systolic blood pressure [SBP] minus diastolic blood pressure [DBP]) is proportional to SV, with variability in the arterial pressure identified as a standard deviation (SD), as indicated in the figure below.

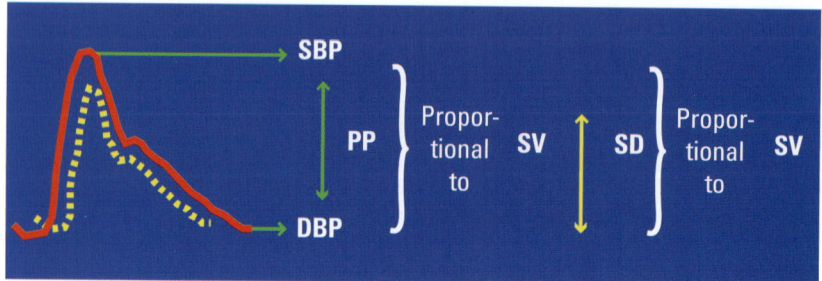

APCO uses a patient's existing arterial catheter to continuously calculate and display CO. The arterial waveform is analyzed by one of three methods (described below) to track changes in SV and CO. Each method uses a different clinically validated algorithm to determine the patient's CO.

- **Pulse flow and pressure analysis:**
  - uses pulse contour and pulse power analysis.
  - incorporates an SD of the full waveform to measure SV.

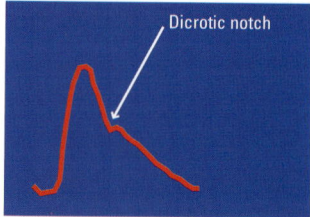

- **Pulse contour analysis:**
  - measures and monitors SV on a beat-to-beat basis looking at the morphology of the arterial waveform from the beginning of systole to the dicrotic notch.

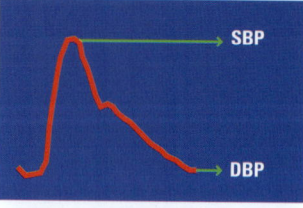

- **Pulse power analysis:**
  - looks at the power of the whole pulse—systolic and diastolic.
  - does not look at beat morphology.

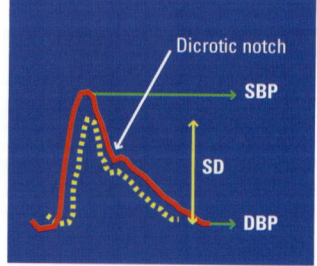

A closer look at APCO monitoring

The arterial catheter (see the figure below) and line are connected to a sensor, transducer, and specialized monitor preprogrammed with the clinically validated algorithm for determining CO.

Three devices are currently available. One system requires that the patient's age, gender, height, and weight be entered into the computer, but no external calibration. Two other systems require an external calibration method. APCO is very useful in helping to determine a patient's fluid status and their potential response to a fluid challenge before they have significant changes in blood pressure.

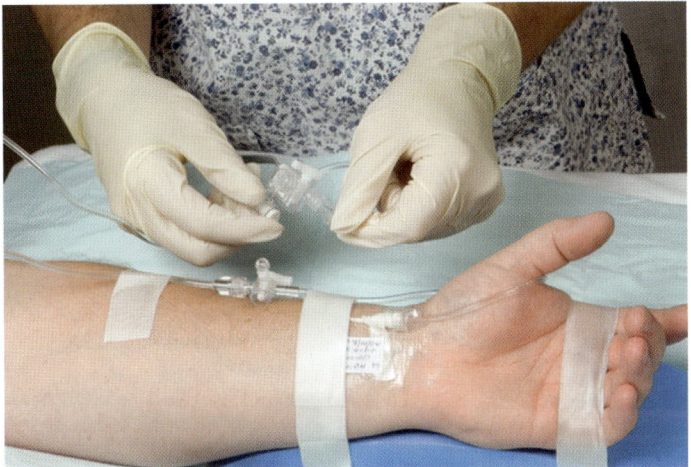

Interfering factors for APCO

• Incorrect leveling of transducer and sensor
• Incorrect zeroing
• IABP
• Arrhythmias
• Artificial heart or ventricular assist device
• Dampened pressure waveforms
• Air bubbles in the fluid line
• Limitations of APCO monitoring: Less accurate with changes in vascular tone and reactivity.

Impedance cardiography

Impedance cardiography provides a noninvasive alternative for tracking hemodynamic status. This technique provides information about a patient's CI, preload, afterload, contractility, CO, and blood flow by measuring low-level electricity that flows harmlessly through the body from electrodes placed on the patient's thorax. These electrodes detect signals elicited from the changing volume and velocity of blood flow through the aorta. The signals are interpreted by the impedance monitor as a waveform. CO is computed from this waveform and the electrocardiogram (ECG).

A closer look at the monitoring equipment for impedance cardiography

To begin impedance cardiography, assemble the impedance cardiography monitor, printer, and disposable sensors.

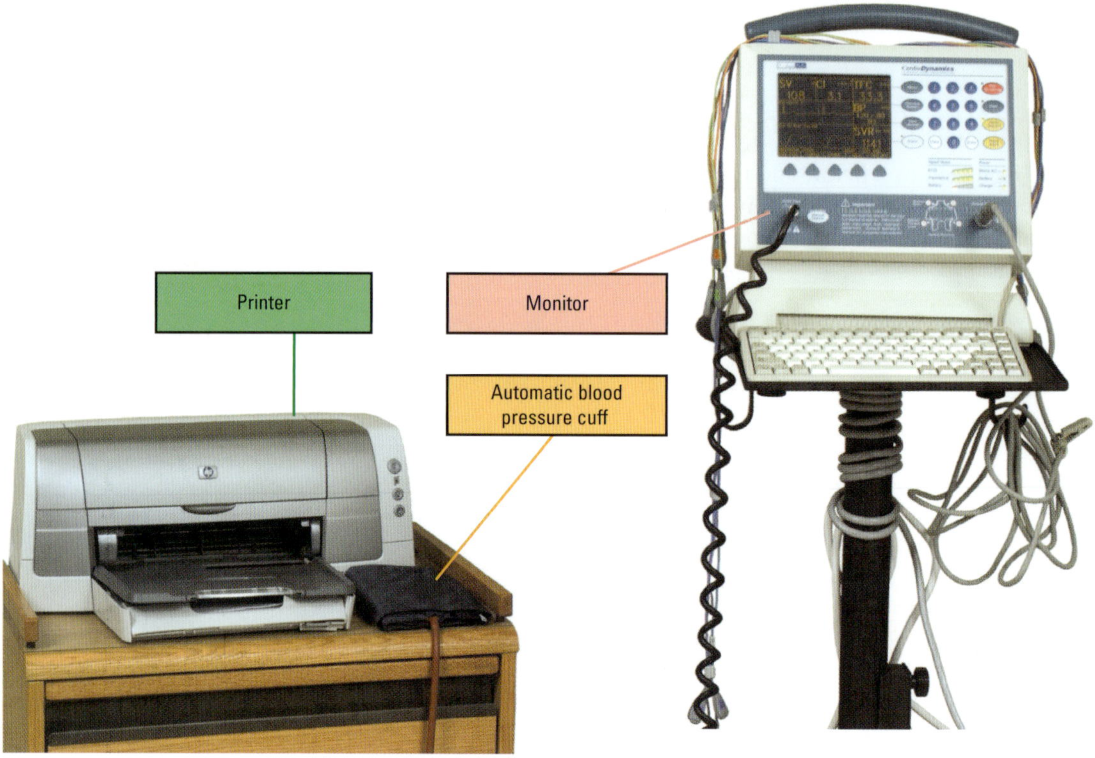

Printer

Monitor

Automatic blood pressure cuff

Benefits of impedance cardiography

Impedance cardiography monitoring eliminates the risk of infection, bleeding, pneumothorax, emboli, and arrhythmias associated with traditional invasive hemodynamic monitoring. The accuracy of results obtained by this method is comparable to that obtained by thermodilution. In addition, the impedance cardiography monitor automatically updates information every 2nd to 10th heartbeat, providing real-time data.

Indications for impedance cardiography

Impedance cardiography helps monitor patients who would have a high risk of complications from thermodilution methods. Because of its portability, the impedance cardiography unit may be used in the operating room, postanesthesia care unit, and intensive care unit.

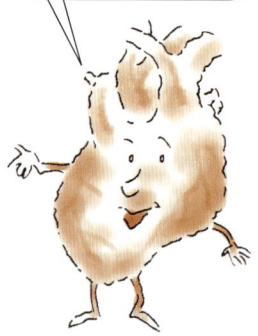

Impedance cardiography is harmless and noninvasive. So there's nothing to *impede* you from using it.

However, baseline impedance cardiography values may be reduced in patients who have conditions characterized by increased fluid in the chest, such as pulmonary edema and pulmonary effusion. Also, impedance cardiography values may be lower than thermodilution values in patients with tachycardia and other arrhythmias.

Impedance cardiography electrode placement

The illustration below and the photograph on the next page show proper placement of the four pairs of electrodes needed for impedance cardiography. This system uses a low-voltage current to detect resistance (impedance) to the current between electrodes.

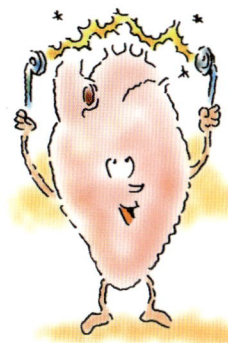

Impedance cardiography uses a low-voltage electric current to detect resistance, or impedance, to the current between the electrodes.

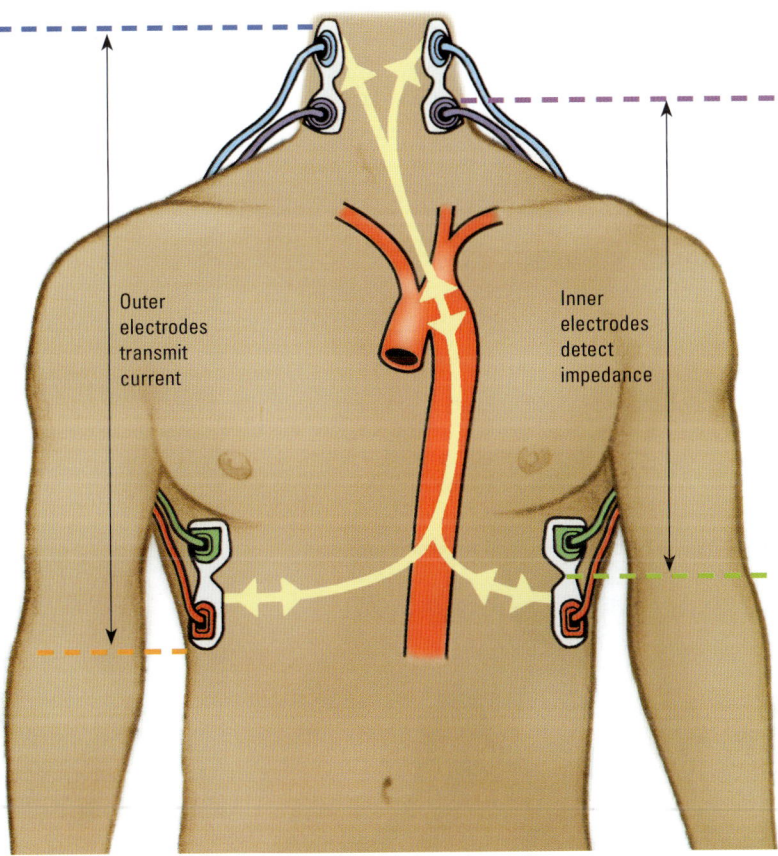

Outer electrodes transmit current

Inner electrodes detect impedance

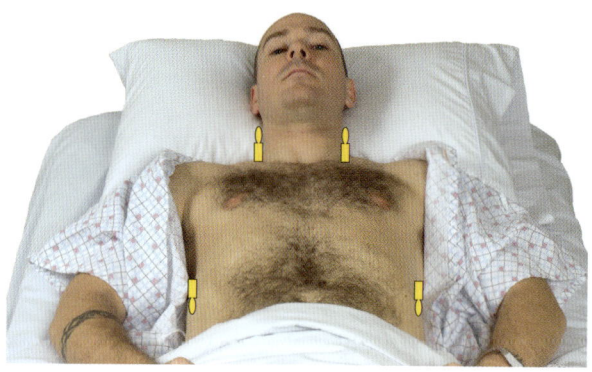
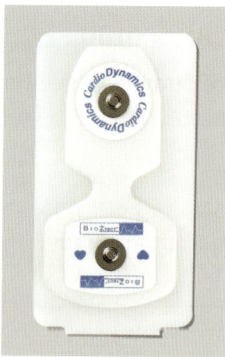

Preparing the patient for impedance cardiography

To prepare a patient for impedance cardiography:

1. Help them into the proper position. The patient should be supine, with the head of the bed elevated at or below 20 degrees.
2. Clean the skin on each side of the neck and on both sides of the chest at the midaxillary line directly across from the xiphoid process using gauze and warm water. Shaving may be necessary to promote adhesion of the electrodes.
3. Hold the patient cable so that the torso diagram is upright and facing you, as shown in the photograph to the right.
4. Connect the leads from top to bottom, following the "BPGO" order (see photograph at bottom right):
    ♦ blue
    ♦ purple
    ♦ green
    ♦ orange.
5. Attach the blood pressure cuff to the patient's arm.

The patient is now ready for impedance cardiography monitoring.

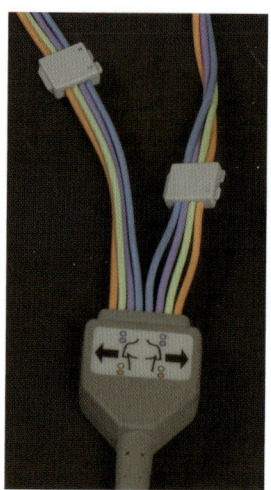

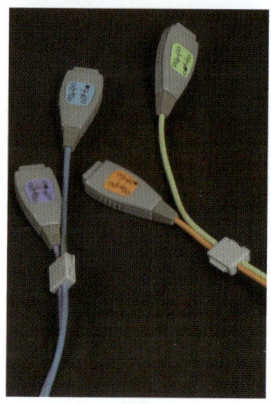

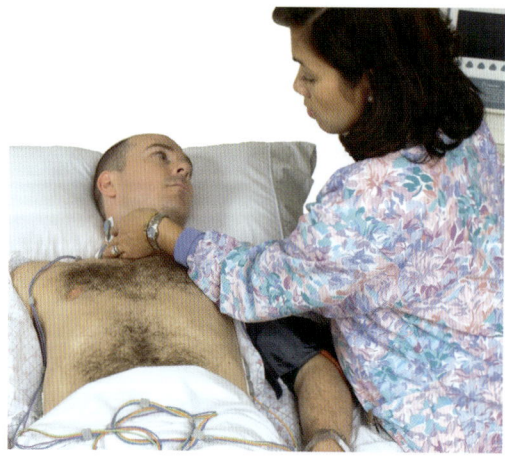

Using the impedance cardiography monitor

To use the impedance cardiography monitor:

1. Plug it in and turn on the power. The welcome display screen should appear.
2. If necessary, enter the basic patient data as prompted by the monitor. The START MONITORING screen should appear.
3. Before initiating monitoring, advise your patient to remain still. Then press the START MONITORING key. Evaluate the signal strength on the screen to make sure that at least three green lights appear on the impedance cardiography and ECG signal bars. In addition, a beep should be audible as each R wave appears on the ECG screen.

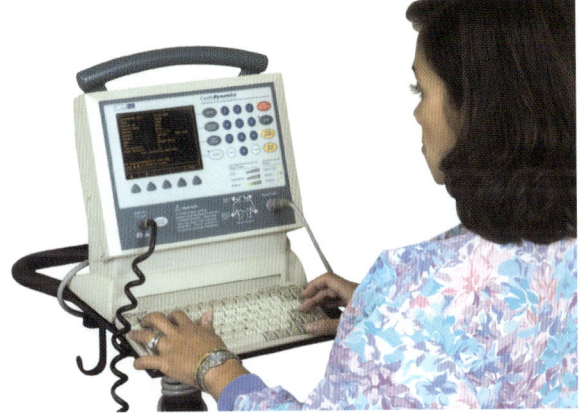
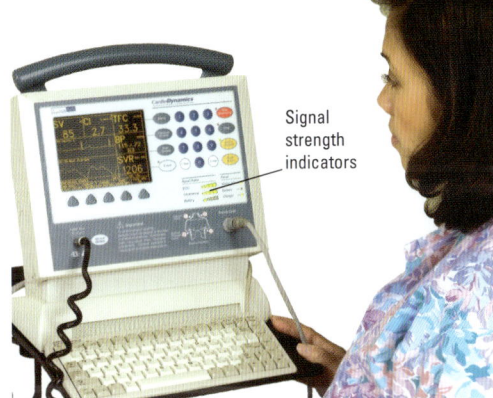

Signal strength indicators

4. Note the waveforms and values on the monitor, and document the values by printing a report.

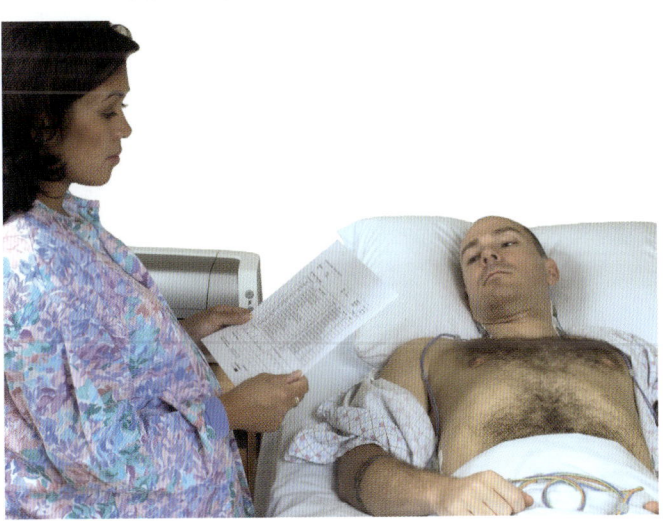

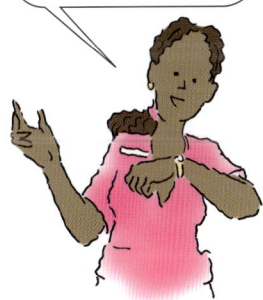

Electrodes should be replaced every 24 hours during continuous impedance cardiography monitoring.

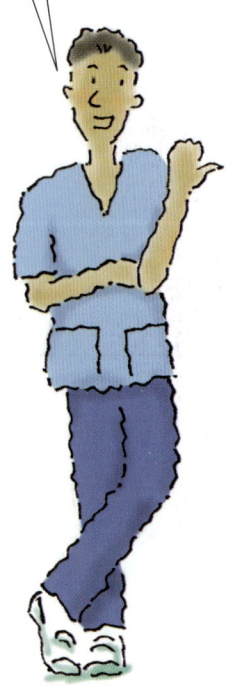

Look at all these indices! Just shows how valuable a tool impedance cardiography is for hemodynamic monitoring!

Understanding hemodynamic indices

After you connect your patient to an impedance cardiography monitor, you can easily obtain the hemodynamic data needed to determine the patient's stability and plan treatment and care. With an impedance cardiography monitoring unit, you can measure these values:

- **Cardiac index:** CO divided by body surface area, which puts CO in perspective for the patient's size
- **Cardiac output:** The volume of blood pumped through the heart (measured in L/min)
- **dZ/dt:** Indicator of peak flow
- **Ejection fraction (EF):** Volume of blood ejected from the left ventricle in a single myocardial contraction (expressed as a percentage)
- **End-diastolic volume (EDV):** Volume of blood in the left ventricle at the end of diastole; also known as the *preload volume* (measured in milliliters)
- **Heart rate:** Number of heartbeats in 1 minute
- **Left cardiac work index (LCWI):** Reflection of myocardial oxygen consumption
- **Pre-ejection period (PEP):** Time between the onset of ventricular activity and the opening of the aortic valve (measured in seconds)
- **Stroke volume:** Amount of blood pumped from the ventricle with each myocardial contraction (measured in milliliters)
- **Systemic vascular resistance:** Resistance against which the left ventricle pumps
- **Ventricular ejection time (VET):** Amount of time that blood is flowing out of the ventricles
- **Zo:** Base impedance, or the amount of resistance met by the electric current passing through the thorax.

Follow the wave

Understanding the impedance cardiography waveform

A waveform produced by an arterial pressure monitoring system is based on pressure. Although a waveform produced by impedance cardiography is similar, it is based on the volume and velocity of aortic blood flow. It captures the electrical impedance of pulsatile flow that is generated by every heartbeat.

The components of an impedance cardiography waveform are shown in the figure below.

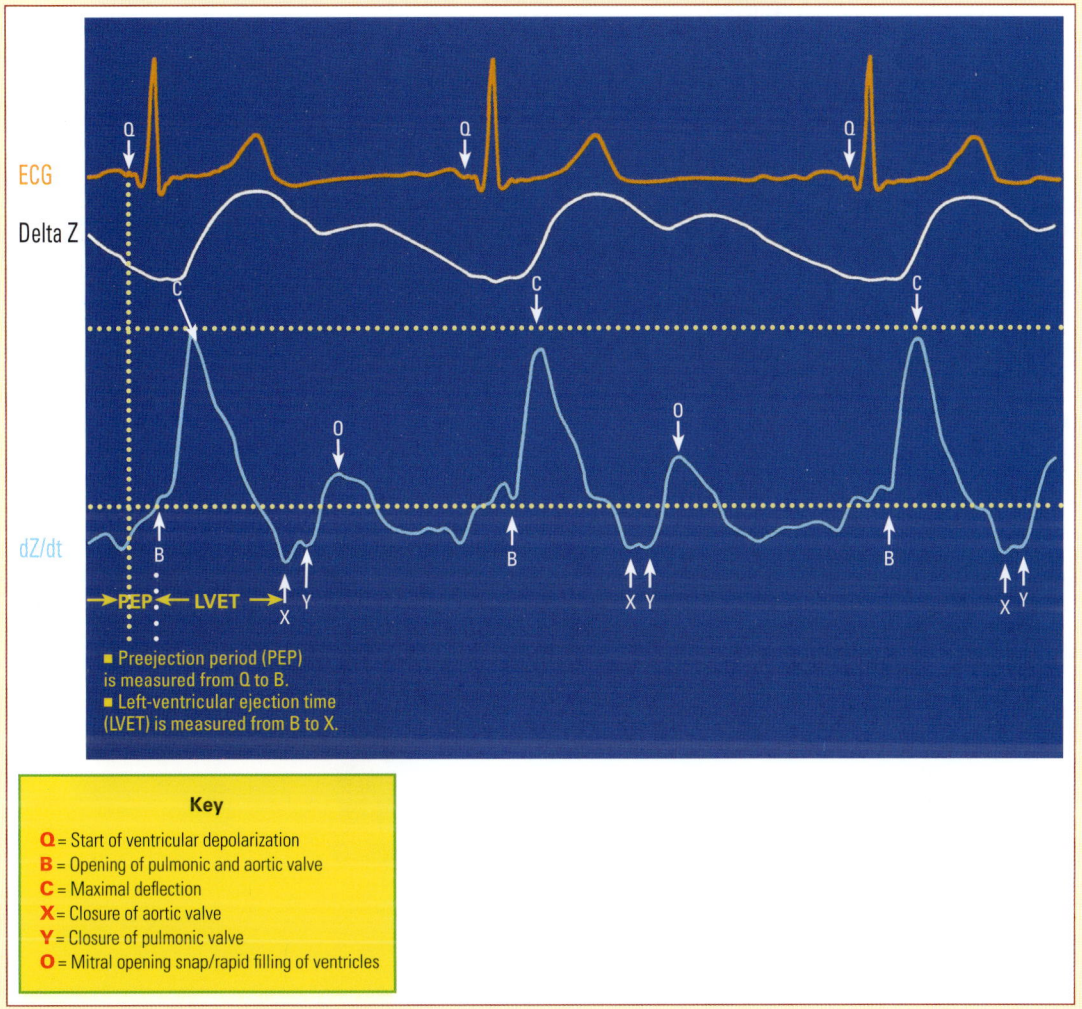

ECG

Delta Z

dZ/dt

■ Preejection period (PEP) is measured from Q to B.
■ Left-ventricular ejection time (LVET) is measured from B to X.

Key
Q = Start of ventricular depolarization
B = Opening of pulmonic and aortic valve
C = Maximal deflection
X = Closure of aortic valve
Y = Closure of pulmonic valve
O = Mitral opening snap/rapid filling of ventricles

The following factors influence correct measurements:
- Incorrect lead placement
- Incorrect patient positioning
- Arrhythmias such as atrial fibrillation
- Weight >351 lb
- Acute aortic insufficiency
- Advanced sepsis
- IABP
- Extreme tachycardia.

Ultrasound CO measurement

Ultrasound cardiac output measurement (USCOM), a technology developed by USCOM Limited in the early 2000s, uses continuous wave Doppler ultrasound to evaluate heart function. This entirely noninvasive system directs the Doppler ultrasound at two anatomic areas:

- The suprasternal notch, to evaluate the left side of the heart by looking at aortic valve blood flow
- The left sternal edge, to evaluate the right side of the heart by looking at pulmonic valve blood flow. Parameters measured by USCOM include CO, CI, SV, HR, velocity time integral, minute distance, ejection time percent, peak flow velocity, and mean pressure gradient.

A closer look at an USCOM monitor

This illustration displays the work screen of a USCOM monitor.

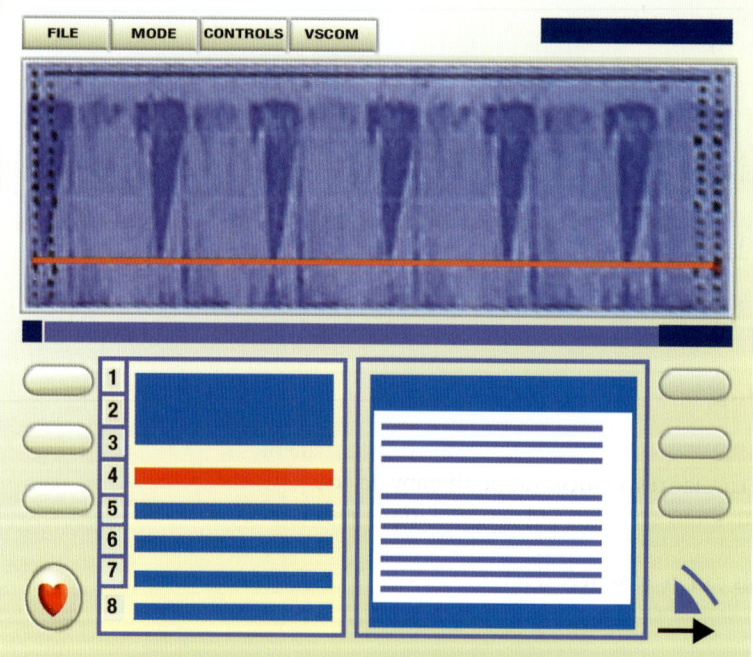

Limitations of this technology include:

- High CO
- Low sedation
- Physiologic structural changes
- Technical and operator factors using echocardiography.

Cardiac bioimpedance

Cardiac bioimpedance can be used to determine hemodynamic parameters including SV, CO, and thoracic fluid content. Change in impedance is measured by alternating current applied across the thorax to determine various hemodynamic parameters. Hemodynamic parameters show changes up to 3 weeks before a heart failure hospitalization. The readings obtained through this technology are used as a guide to optimize heart failure therapy.

ReDS vest by Sensible Medical is a wearable vest that quantifies the amount of lung fluid noninvasively through radar technology. ReDS stands for remote dielectric sensing. A specialized vest is applied to the patient, and a reading is obtained within 45 seconds. It is usually used in an outpatient setting and is noninvasive.

Limitations of cardiac bioimpedance technology include:
- Not continuous
- Accuracy is user dependent.

Patients excluded in cardiac bioimpedance technology include those with any of the following characteristics:
- Height <155 cm or >190 cm
- BMI <22 or >39
- Chest circumference <80 cm, >115 cm, or flail chest
- Focal lung lesions—active pneumonia, pulmonary emboli, known lung nodule, lung carcinoma
- Renal failure
- Cardiac surgery within 2 months
- Left ventricular assist device (LVAD) or cardiac transplant
- Congenital heart malformations such as dextrocardia.

Electrophysiology with fluid monitoring in pacemakers

If a patient with heart failure meets criteria for a biventricular permanent pacemaker (PPM) or a cardiac resynchronization therapy device, several device options that incorporate fluid accumulation detection are available. Rise in fluid accumulation will trigger an alert for the electrophysiologist. This can be remotely monitored along with a pacemaker report.

Examples include:
- OptiVol fluid status monitoring is a system within Medtronic implantable cardioverter-defibrillator devices and cardiac resynchronization therapy with defibrillator. The OptiVol system trends and tracks intrathoracic impedance changes over time to guide medical therapy. The SENSE-HF trial showed low sensitivity in the early period after implanting the device, which improved over the 6 months following implant.

- HeartLogic Heart Failure Diagnostic-Heart Failure Management System within implantable cardioverter-defibrillator devices uses five physiologic sensors (heart sounds, thoracic impedance, respiration, HR, and activity) to track physiologic trends and combines them into one composite index, which is a mathematical equation as an algorithm. It has 70% sensitivity and can detect a heart failure event up to 34 days prior. If the index rises above the threshold (>16), it will send proactive alerts of potential worsening heart failure.

CardioMEMS

The CardioMEMS system is an implanted sensor placed in the distal PA during a right heart catheterization through a venous access; therefore, no contrast that could cause damage to the kidneys is needed. The sensor is simply a sensor, and it is paired with a pillow the patient lies on that includes a wand that is powered by radio-frequency energy. PA pressures and HR are transmitted wirelessly to an online portal that can be accessed by the health care team. (See https://www.cardiovascular.abbott/cardiomemsisw for more information about this system.)

PA pressure changes begin a few days to weeks before the onset of overt heart failure symptoms. Monitoring of these pressures and changes enables modification of the heart failure treatment plan to reduce heart failure hospitalizations by adjusting the patient's diuretics. HR is also monitored, which could pick up rapid arrhythmias. This technology can be used for all types and etiologies of heart failure.

Quick quiz

Color my world

Use a green pen or pencil to trace the proper placement of a transesophageal Doppler probe in the illustration.

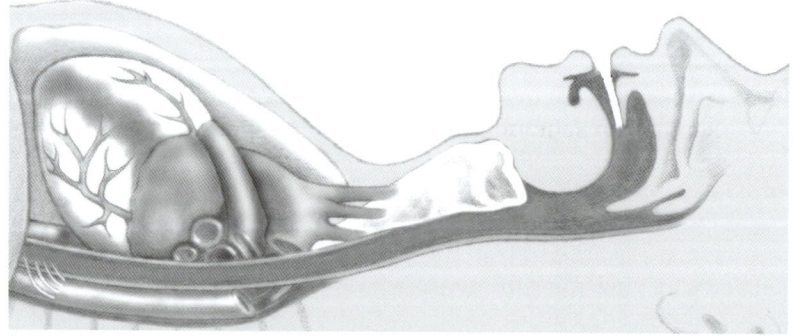

Picture imperfect

Identify the picture that shows the correct electrode placement for impedance cardiography.

1.

2.

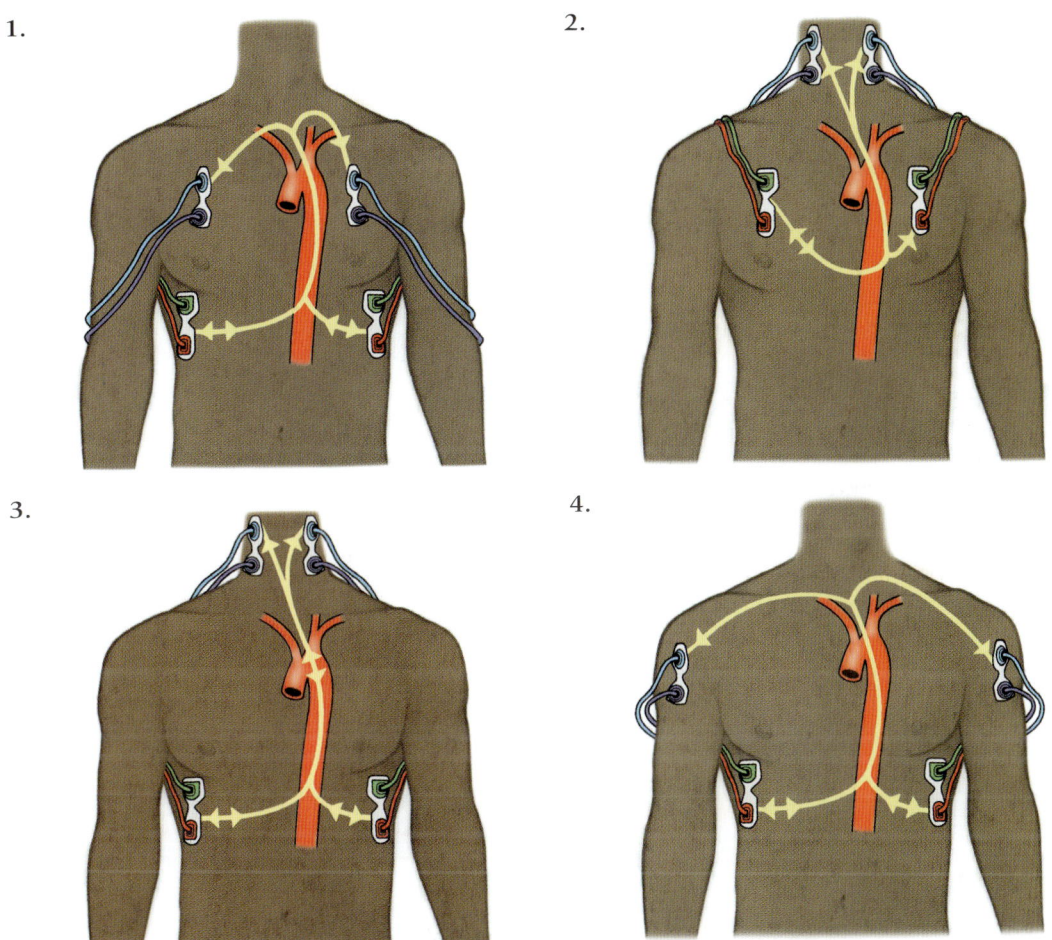

3.

4.

ment is shown in #3.
esophagus, posterior to the heart; Picture imperfect: Correct electrode place-
orally to the appropriate depth marker. The tip of the probe should lie in the
Answers: Color my world: After lubricating the tube, insert it either nasally or

Selected references

Ancha, S., Auberle, C., Cash, D., Harsh, M., Hickman, J., & Kounga, C. (Eds.). (2023). *Washington manual of medical therapeutics* (37th ed.). Lippincott Williams & Wilkins.

Berndsen, M. (2022). Non-invasive and minimally invasive cardiac output monitoring a nursing perspective. *Dimensions of Critical Care Nursing, 41*(3), 121–123. https://doi.org/10.1097/DCC.0000000000000524

Bodys-Pelka, A., Kusztal, M., Boszko, M., Główczyńska, R., & Grabowski, M. (2021). Non-invasive measurement for haemodynamic parameters-clinical utility. *Journal of Clinical Medicine, 10*(21), 4929. https://doi.org/10.3390/jcm10214929

Johnson, K. (2023). *AACN procedure manual for progressive and critical care* (8th ed.). Elsevier.

Chapter 10

Circulatory assist devices

Understanding circulatory assist devices

Circulatory assist devices support or aid the heart's pumping ability in patients with heart failure. These devices improve blood flow to the myocardium and the rest of the body while reducing myocardial workload.

Such devices include intra-aortic balloon pump (IABP) counterpulsation; ventricular assist devices (VADs), including percutaneous VADs such as the Impella; and extracorporeal membrane oxygenation (ECMO).

Intra-aortic balloon pump counterpulsation

Providing temporary support for the heart's left ventricle, IABP counterpulsation mechanically displaces blood within the aorta by means of an intra-aortic balloon attached to an external pump console. The balloon is usually inserted through the common femoral artery and positioned with its tip just distal to the left subclavian artery. When used correctly, IABP improves two key aspects of myocardial physiology: It increases the supply of oxygen-rich blood to the myocardium and decreases myocardial oxygen demand.

Insertion of the intra–aortic balloon

The following figure explains the steps to insert an intra-aortic balloon.

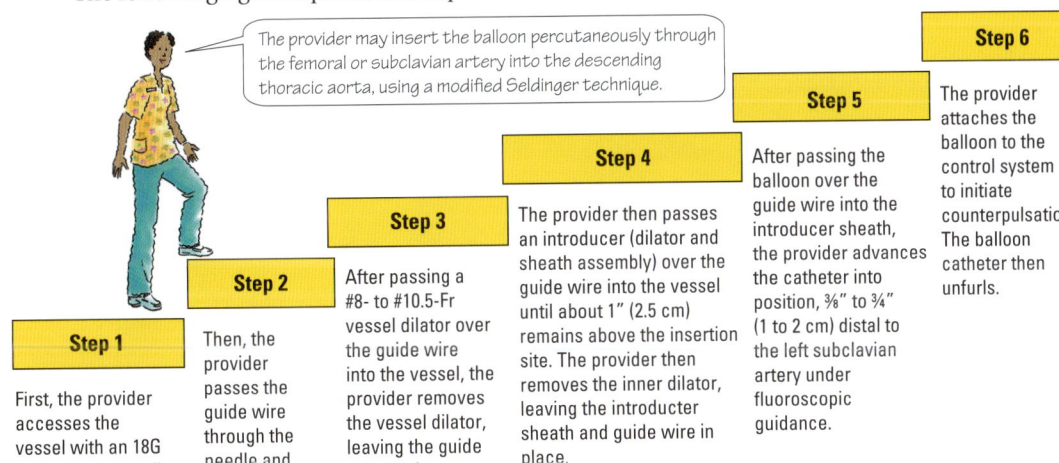

The provider may insert the balloon percutaneously through the femoral or subclavian artery into the descending thoracic aorta, using a modified Seldinger technique.

Step 1

First, the provider accesses the vessel with an 18G angiography needle and removes the inner stylet.

Step 2

Then, the provider passes the guide wire through the needle and removes the needle.

Step 3

After passing a #8- to #10.5-Fr vessel dilator over the guide wire into the vessel, the provider removes the vessel dilator, leaving the guide wire in place.

Step 4

The provider then passes an introducer (dilator and sheath assembly) over the guide wire into the vessel until about 1" (2.5 cm) remains above the insertion site. The provider then removes the inner dilator, leaving the introducer sheath and guide wire in place.

Step 5

After passing the balloon over the guide wire into the introducer sheath, the provider advances the catheter into position, ⅜" to ¾" (1 to 2 cm) distal to the left subclavian artery under fluoroscopic guidance.

Step 6

The provider attaches the balloon to the control system to initiate counterpulsation. The balloon catheter then unfurls.

141

Indications and contraindications for intra-aortic balloon pump counterpulsation

IABP counterpulsation is recommended for patients with:

- refractory anginas.
- ventricular arrhythmias associated with ischemia.
- pump failure caused by cardiogenic shock, intraoperative myocardial infarction (MI), or low cardiac output after bypass surgery.
- low cardiac output secondary to acute mechanical defects after MI (such as ventricular septal defect, papillary muscle rupture, or left ventricular aneurysm).
- a suspected high-grade lesion (used perioperatively for those who are undergoing such procedures as angioplasty, thrombolytic therapy, cardiac surgery, and cardiac catheterization).

IABP counterpulsation is contraindicated in patients with:

- severe aortic insufficiency.
- aortic aneurysm.
- severe peripheral vascular disease.

Surgical insertion sites for the intra-aortic balloon

If an intra-aortic balloon cannot be inserted percutaneously, the provider will insert it surgically, using a femoral or transthoracic approach.

Femoral approach

Insertion through the femoral artery requires a cutdown and an arteriotomy. The provider passes the balloon through a Dacron graft that has been sewn to the artery.

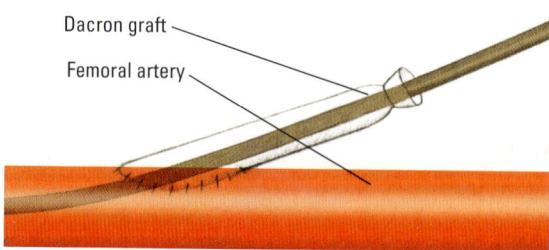

Dacron graft

Femoral artery

Subclavian approach

Insertion through the subclavian artery is done under fluoroscopic guidance; the balloon wire is positioned in the descending thoracic aorta, and the balloon is inserted and placed in an appropriate position.

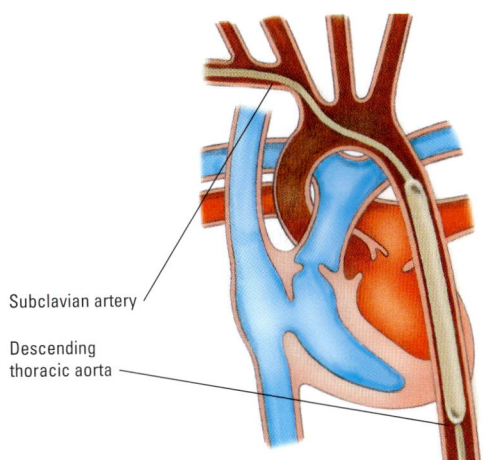

Subclavian artery

Descending thoracic aorta

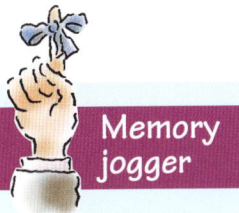

Memory jogger

To remember what happens when using an IABP, think of these pictures.

Transthoracic approach

If femoral insertion is unsuccessful, the provider may use a transthoracic approach. The provider inserts the balloon in an antegrade direction through the subclavian artery and then positions it in the descending thoracic aorta.

How the intra-aortic balloon pump works

Made of polyurethane, the intra-aortic balloon is attached to an external pump console by means of a large-lumen catheter. The illustrations in this section show the direction of blood flow when the pump inflates and deflates the balloon.

Balloon inflation

The balloon inflates as the aortic valve closes and diastole begins. During diastole, the balloon inflates, sending blood back to the heart, which then increases perfusion to the coronary arteries.

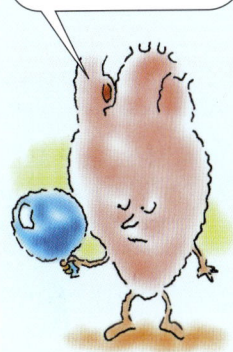

During balloon inflation, perfusion to the coronary arteries is increased.

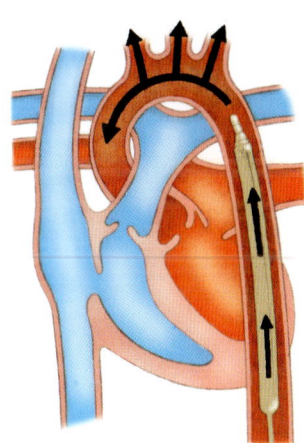

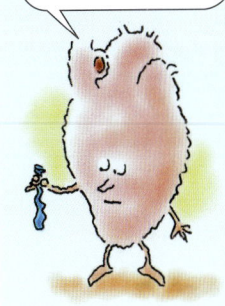

During balloon deflation, aortic end-diastolic pressure and afterload are decreased.

Balloon deflation

The balloon deflates before ventricular ejection, when the aortic valve opens. This deflation permits ejection of blood from the left ventricle against a lowered resistance. As a result, aortic end-diastolic pressure and afterload decrease and cardiac output rises.

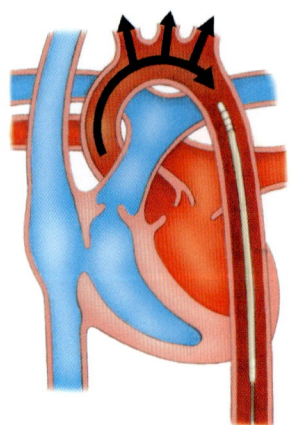

Normal inflation–deflation timing

Balloon inflation occurs after aortic valve closure; deflation occurs during isovolumetric contraction, just before the aortic valve opens. In a properly timed waveform such as this one, the inflation point lies at or slightly above the dicrotic notch. Both inflation and deflation cause a sharp V. Peak diastolic pressure exceeds peak systolic pressure; peak systolic pressure exceeds assisted peak systolic pressure.

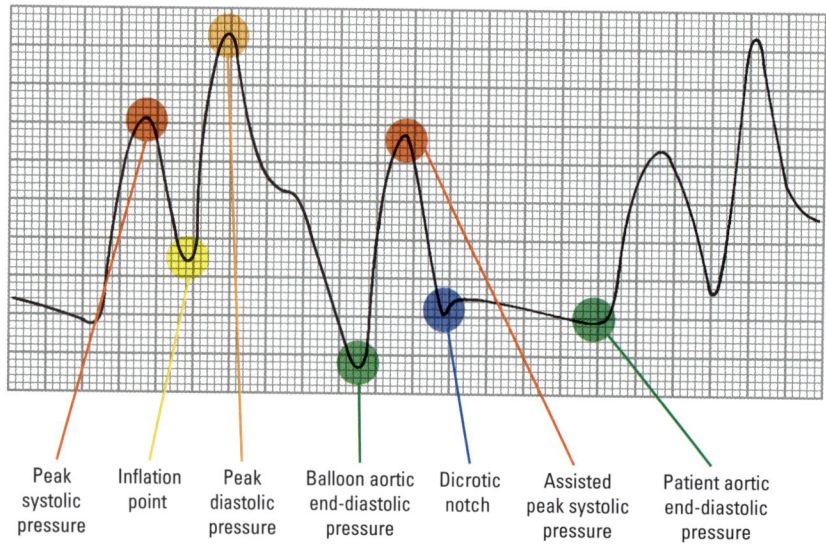

Peak systolic pressure   Inflation point   Peak diastolic pressure   Balloon aortic end-diastolic pressure   Dicrotic notch   Assisted peak systolic pressure   Patient aortic end-diastolic pressure

Early inflation

With early inflation, the inflation point lies before the dicrotic notch. Early inflation dangerously increases myocardial stress and decreases cardiac output.

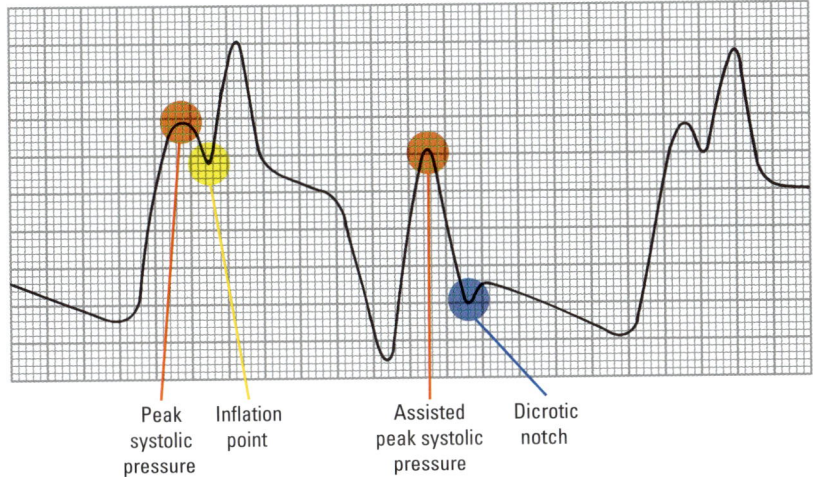

Peak systolic pressure   Inflation point   Assisted peak systolic pressure   Dicrotic notch

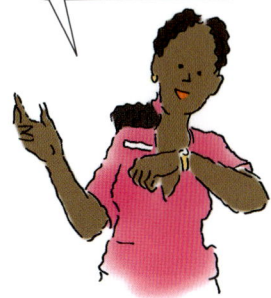

With IABP, timing is everything. Early or late inflation or deflation can endanger the patient. Check out these waveforms to learn how to spot IABP problems!

Early deflation

With early deflation, a U shape appears, and peak systolic pressure is less than or equal to assisted peak systolic pressure. Early deflation won't decrease afterload or myocardial oxygen consumption.

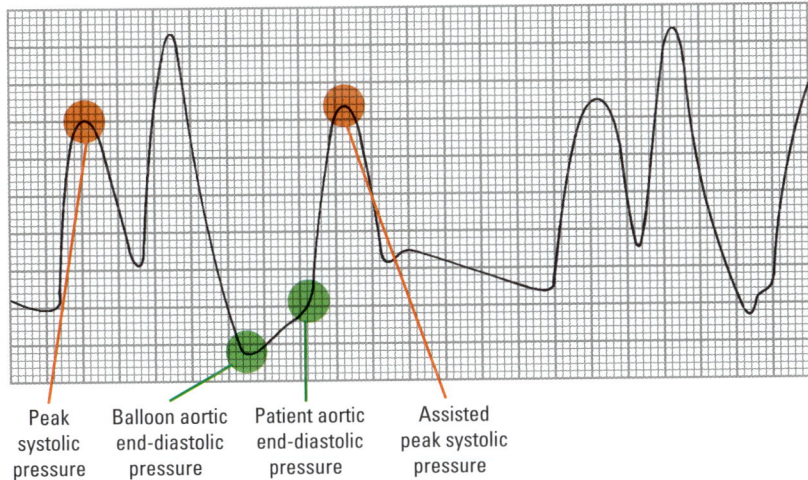

Peak systolic pressure   Balloon aortic end-diastolic pressure   Patient aortic end-diastolic pressure   Assisted peak systolic pressure

Late inflation

With late inflation, the dicrotic notch precedes the inflation point, and the notch and the inflation point create a W shape. Late inflation can lead to a reduction in peak diastolic pressure, coronary and systemic perfusion augmentation time, and augmented coronary perfusion pressure.

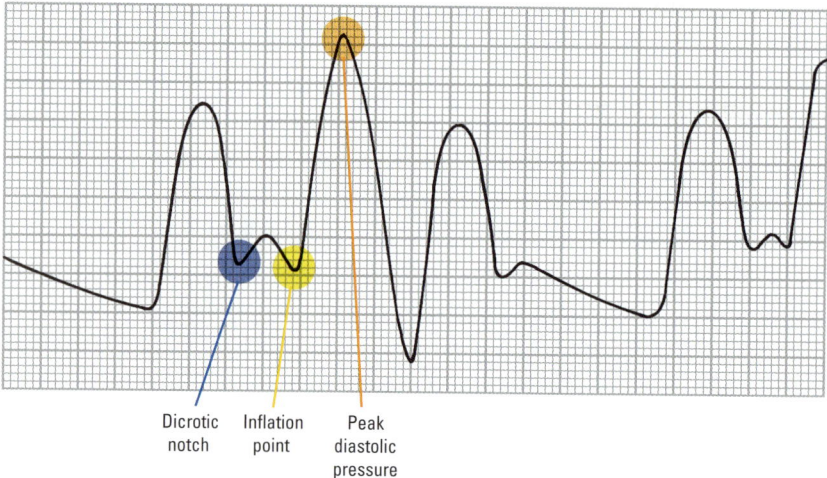

Dicrotic notch   Inflation point   Peak diastolic pressure

Late deflation

With late deflation, peak systolic pressure exceeds assisted peak systolic pressure. Late deflation puts the patient at risk by increasing afterload, myocardial oxygen consumption, cardiac workload, and preload.

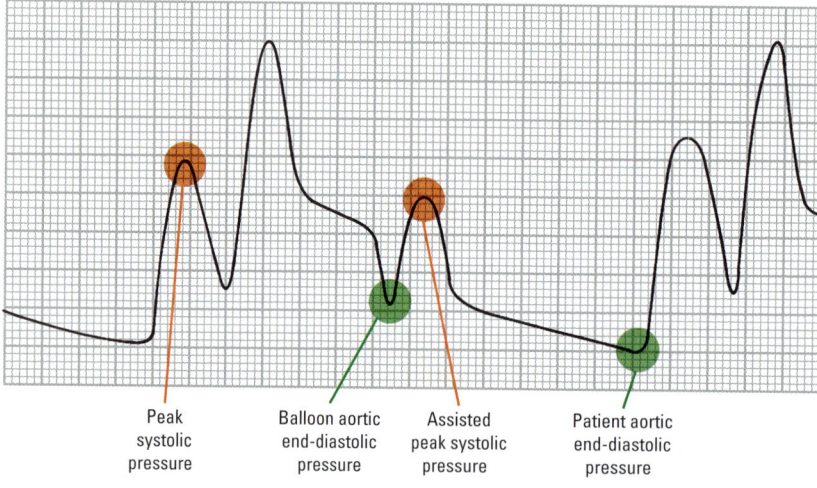

Peak systolic pressure   Balloon aortic end-diastolic pressure   Assisted peak systolic pressure   Patient aortic end-diastolic pressure

Follow the wave

Heart rate and blood pressure effects on intra-aortic balloon pump waveforms

Changes in heart rate and blood pressure cause changes in the width and height of the balloon pressure plateau of the IABP waveform, as shown in the following illustrations.

Changes in heart rate

Variations in heart rate affect the width of the balloon pressure plateau. Note: If the width of the balloon pressure plateau is not consistent with the patient's heart rate, there may be a significant error in timing.

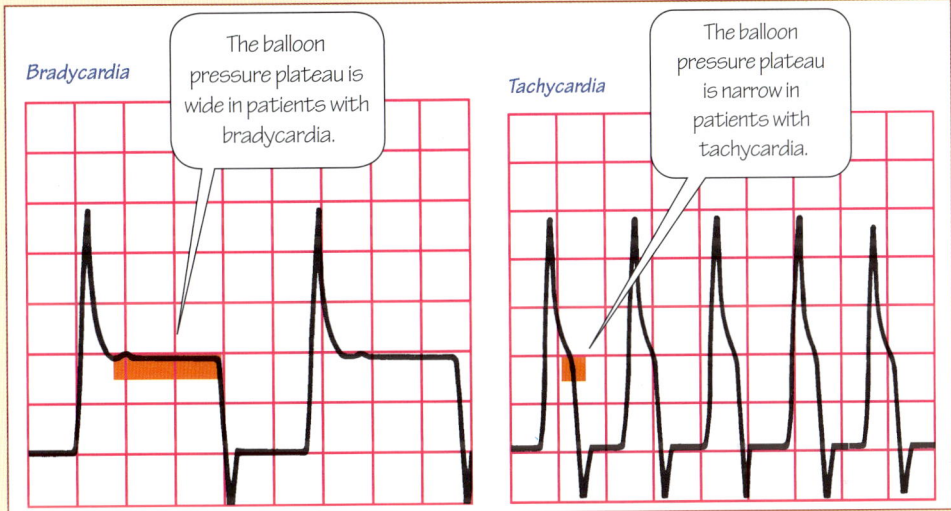

Changes in blood pressure

Variations in blood pressure affect the height of the balloon pressure plateau.

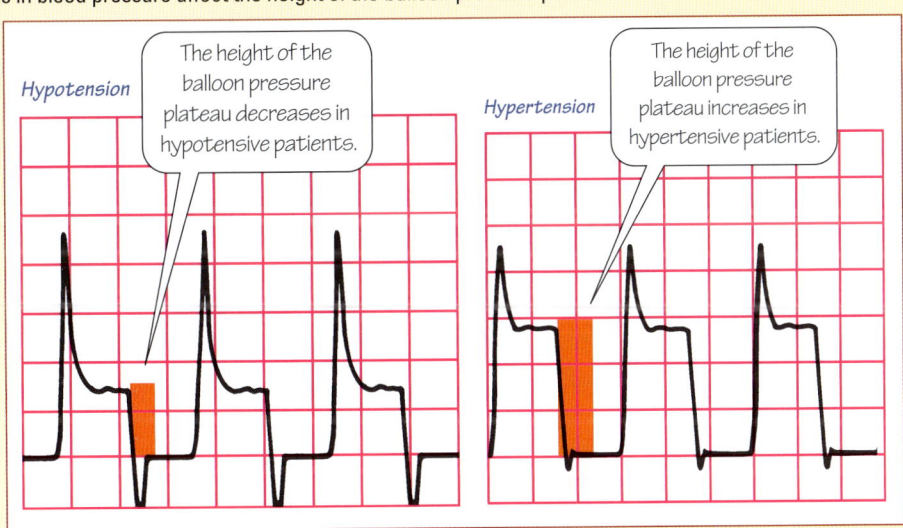

Complications of intra–aortic balloon pump counterpulsation

IABP counterpulsation may cause numerous complications. The most common—arterial embolism—stems from clot formation on the balloon surface. Other potential complications include extension or rupture of an aortic aneurysm, visceral and limb ischemia, femoral or iliac artery perforation, femoral artery occlusion, and sepsis. Bleeding at the insertion site may result from pump-induced thrombocytopenia.

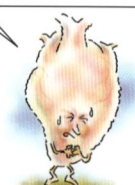

Arterial embolism is the most common complication of IABP counterpulsation.

 **Follow the wave**

Abnormal intra-aortic balloon pump waveforms

The below table describes some abnormal IABP waveforms and their causes.

Abnormality	Waveform	Causes
Low balloon pressure plateau		• Hypotension • Hypovolemia • Low systemic vascular resistance • Balloon that is too small for the aorta or low balloon inflation volume • Positioning of balloon too low in aorta
High balloon pressure plateau		• Hypertension • Balloon that is too large for the aorta • Restriction of gas flow in the system
Balloon pressure baseline elevation		• Restriction of gas flow • Overpressurized gas in the system
Balloon pressure baseline depression		• Helium leak • Inappropriate timing settings • Mechanical defect

Troubleshooting an intra-aortic balloon pump

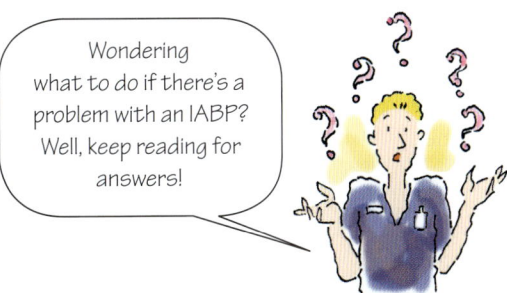

Wondering what to do if there's a problem with an IABP? Well, keep reading for answers!

Problem	Possible causes	Interventions
High gas leak (automatic mode only)	Balloon leakage or abrasion	• Check for blood in the tubing. • Stop pumping. • Notify the provider to remove the balloon.
	Condensation in extension tubing, volume limiter disk, or both	• Remove condensate from the tubing and volume limiter disk. • Refill, autopurge, and resume pumping.
	Kink in a balloon catheter or tubing	• Check the catheter and tubing for kinks and loose connections; straighten and tighten any found. • Refill and resume pumping.
	Tachycardia	• Change wean control to 1:2 or operate on "manual" mode. • Autopurge the balloon every 1–2 hours and monitor the balloon pressure waveform closely.
	Malfunctioning or loose volume limiter disk	• Replace or tighten the disk. • Refill, autopurge, and resume pumping.
	System leak	• Perform a leak test.
Balloon line block (in automatic mode only)	Kink in a balloon or catheter	• Check the catheter and tubing for kinks and loose connections; straighten and tighten any found. • Refill and resume pumping.
	Balloon catheter not unfurled; sheath or balloon positioned too high	• Notify the provider immediately to verify placement. • Anticipate the need for repositioning or manual inflation of the balloon.
	Condensation in tubing, volume limiter disk, or both	• Remove condensate from the tubing and volume limiter disk. • Refill, autopurge, and resume pumping.
	Balloon too large for aorta	• Decrease the volume control percentage by one notch.
	Malfunctioning volume limiter disk or incorrect volume limiter disk size	• Replace the volume limiter disk. • Refill, autopurge, and resume pumping.
No electrocardiogram (ECG) trigger	Inadequate signal	• Adjust ECG gain and change the lead or trigger mode.
	Lead disconnected	• Replace the lead.
	Improper ECG input mode (skin or monitor) selected	• Adjust ECG input to appropriate mode (skin or monitor).

Problem	Possible causes	Interventions
No atrial pressure trigger	Arterial line damped	• Flush the line.
	Arterial line open to atmosphere	• Check connections on the arterial pressure line.
Trigger mode change	Trigger mode changed while pumping	• Resume pumping.
Irregular heart rhythm	Patient experiencing arrhythmia, such as atrial fibrillation or ectopic beats	• Change to R or QRS sense (to accommodate irregular rhythm, if necessary). • Notify the provider of arrhythmia.
Erratic atrioventricular (AV) pacing	Demand for paced rhythm occur-ring when in AV sequential trigger mode	• Change to pacer reject trigger or QRS sense.
Noisy ECG signal	Malfunctioning leads	• Replace the leads. • Check the ECG cable.
	Electrocautery in use	• Switch to atrial pressure trigger.
Internal trigger	Trigger mode set on internal 80 beats/min	• Select an alternative trigger if the patient has a heartbeat or rhythm. • Keep in mind that the internal trigger is used only during cardiopulmonary bypass or cardiac arrest.
Purge incomplete	Off button pressed during autopurge; interrupted purge cycle	• Initiate autopurging again, or initiate pumping.
High fill pressure	Malfunctioning volume limiter disk	• Replace the volume limiter disk. • Refill, autopurge, and resume pumping.
	Occluded vent line or valve	• Attempt to resume pumping. • If unsuccessful, notify the provider and contact the manufacturer.
No balloon drive	No volume limiter disk	• Insert the volume limiter disk and lock it securely in place.
	Tubing disconnected	• Reconnect the tubing. • Refill, autopurge, and pump.
Incorrect timing	Inflate and deflate controls set incorrectly	• Place the inflate and deflate controls at set midpoints. • Reassess timing and readjust.
Low volume percentage	Volume control percentage not 100%	• Assess the cause of decreased volume and reset (if necessary).

Ventricular assist devices

Patients with severe ventricular dysfunction, where an IABP would be insufficient, can be supported with a temporary device. This device serves as a bridge to either a heart transplant or a permanent VAD.

Temporary ventricular assist devices

A temporary VAD is a mini, axial flow VAD for temporary hemody-namic support. It sits across the aortic valve, pulls blood from the left ventricle, and ejects the blood into the ascending aorta. The goal of the device is to let the heart rest and recover; it can do the work until hemodynamic recovery is achieved. Indications for use are:

- cardiogenic shock on a short-term basis use to allow the heart to rest/recover; if no recovery, transition to a more durable device
- pre- or post-percutaneous coronary intervention or electrophysiology procedure
- post-op myocardial stunning
- primary graft dysfunction in heart transplant
- left ventricle (LV) vent for ECMO patients

  Contraindications for temporary VAD placement are a mural thrombus in the left ventricle, mechanical aortic valve, aortic valve stenosis or calcification, moderate-to-severe aortic insufficiency, or severe peripheral vascular disease.

Positioning of temporary ventricular assist devices

Placement is confirmed by an echocardiogram. The cannula bend should be at the aortic valve annulus, placing the inlet approximately 5 cm deep into the ventricle. The catheter outlet area sits above the aortic valve. The catheter sits across the aortic valve.

The catheter is angled toward the left ventricle apex away from the heat wall, not curled up or blocking the mitral valve.

Parameters of temporary ventricular assist devices

Power level

Power level (P level) determines the flow of the pump. It is not a linear relationship between power and flow; the flow will vary in each patient based on the P level. The higher the P level, the faster the motor is spinning, and the higher the flow should be.

P-level	Flow rate (L/min) mAP 60-100	*Flow rate (L/min)	Revolutions per minute (rpm)
P-0	0.0	0.0	0
P-1	0.0–0.1	0.0–1.4	10,000
P-2	0.7–2.1	0.5–2.6	17,000
P-3	1.2–2.7	0.5–3.1	20,000
P-4	1.9–3.1	0.9–3.4	22,000
P-5	2.8–3.5	1.4–3.7	24,000
P-6	3.3–3.8	1.8–4.0	26,000
P-7	3.7–4.1	2.6–4.4	28,000
P-8	4.1–4.5	3.4–4.7	30,000
P-9	4.7–5.1	4.2–5.3	33,000

*Flow rate can vary due to suction or incorrect positioning.

Motor current

The motor current indicates how much a temporary VAD motor uses to move blood during systole and diastole. Measured in milliampere (microbe-associated molecular patterns), it does not have a set range; the trend is followed. The motor current rises with increased flows and falls with decreased flows. During systole, when the aortic valve is open, there is an increase in flow; and there is no longer a gradient. When the valve closes during diastole, flow and motor current decrease, and the gradient returns. A pulsatile motor current indicates that the temporary VAD device is properly positioned across the aortic valve.

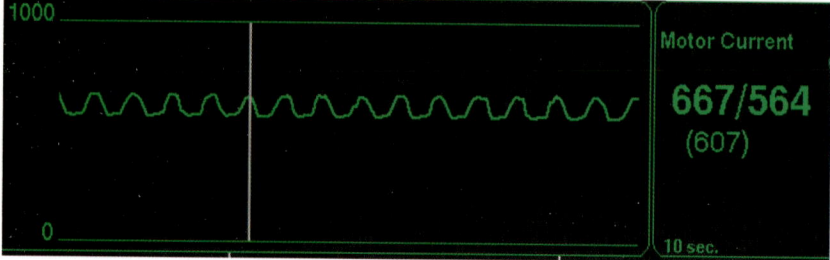

Motor current changes

Flat motor current indicates incorrect positioning, with the inlet and outlet areas in the same chamber without the gradient across the aortic valve. Erratic pulsatile signal can be indicative of suction. As the P level (speed) increases, overall workload increases, which increases the motor current. Motor current can also increase if there is an issue within the purge system and blood gets inside the motor housing. If the motor current increases rapidly, it may be indicative of a clot or impending pump failure.

Placement signal

The placement signal helps determine the correct placement of the catheter. It is a pressure measurement. If the temporary VAD is in the correct position, the placement signal will measure aortic arterial pressure, as shown in this image.

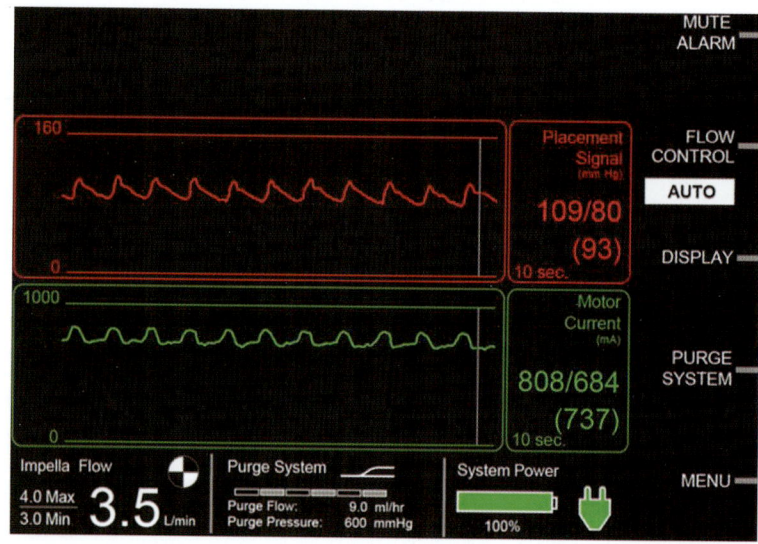

You can't use this as a substitute for arterial line pressure. If the temporary VAD has migrated into the LV, it will look like an LV pressure tracing, as shown below.

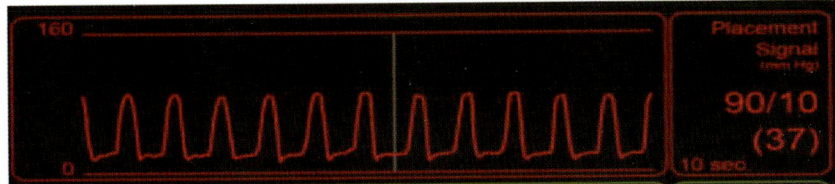

If the temporary VAD has migrated into the aorta, the wave form will look like an arterial wave form, as shown below.

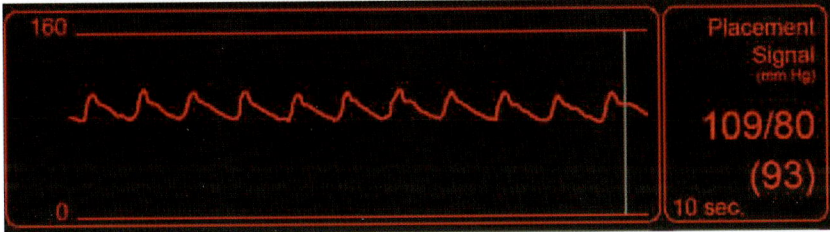

Durable left ventricular assist device

A VAD is implanted to provide support to a (left) failing heart. The device consists of a blood pump, cannulas, and a pneumatic or electrical drive console (or controller). A VAD can provide systemic and pulmonary support.

VADs are designed to decrease the heart's workload and to increase cardiac output in patients with ventricular failure. They are commonly used as a bridge to cardiac transplantation. VADs are also indicated for use in patients with:

- end-stage heart failure, but who are ineligible for a transplant (destination therapy)
- cardiogenic shock that does not respond to maximal pharmacologic therapy
- inability to be weaned from cardiopulmonary bypass.

Insertion of a ventricular assist device

Insertion of a VAD involves a specific surgical procedure—a median sternotomy, in which blood is diverted from a ventricle to an artificial pump. The diversion is created by inserting a cannula into either the atria or ventricles that direct blood to the pump. This pump then functions as the ventricle. An inflow cannula drains blood from the left atrium or ventricle into the VAD, which then pushes the blood into the ascending aorta through the outflow cannula and outflow graft.

Implantable ventricular assist devices

The typical durable VAD (such as HeartMate II and HeartMate 3) is implanted in the upper abdominal wall (HeartMate II) or attached directly to the heart (HeartMate 3). HeartMate II was one of the original VADs, and when it first came out, it was the VAD to implant. However, with newer technology, HeartMate 3 is the only durable VAD being implanted currently. HeartMate II requires a longer bypass time because the surgeon must create a pocket for the pump to sit inside in the patient's abdomen. HeartMate 3 needs a shorter bypass time because the VAD is sewn directly to the patient's pericardium.

Pump options

Continuous flow pump

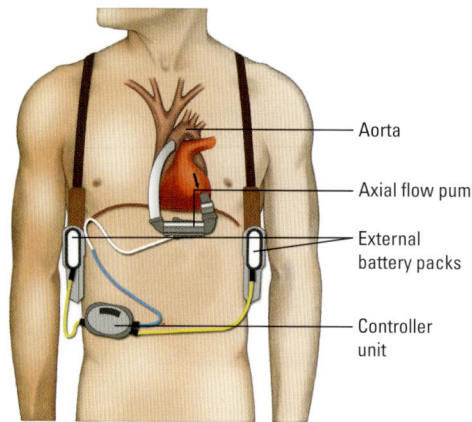

- Aorta
- Axial flow pump
- External battery packs
- Controller unit

Pulsatile pump

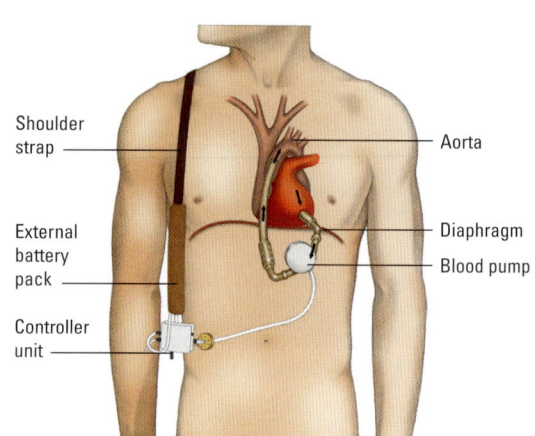

- Shoulder strap
- Aorta
- External battery pack
- Diaphragm
- Blood pump
- Controller unit

VADs are available as continuous flow (CF; axial or centrifugal flow) or pulsatile pumps. A CF pump fills continuously and returns blood to the aorta at a constant rate. CF VADs move blood forward by centrifugal force by a rotating cone (HeartMate 3). CF VADs are nonpulsatile in that the patient's aortic valve is not usually opening, or if it is opening, it is opening every other beat or so. Patients with an ejection fraction of 5% will have some native contribution to the pump. A ventricle that is not contracting at all will allow for stagnant blood and will lead to clot formation. The total artificial heart (TAH) is a pneumatically driven pulsatile pump. The TAH is used for patients with biventricular failure and completely replaces their heart with either two 50- or 70-mL plastic ventricles; the only portion of a patient's native heart that is left is their atrial leaflets. The blood is then moved through the ventricles by the compressed air through four metal valves.

A pulsatile pump may work in one of two ways:

1. It may fill during systole and pump blood into the aorta during diastole.
2. It may pump regardless of the patient's cardiac cycle.

Placing the ventricular assist device

VADs divert blood from failing ventricles to a pump that can effectively eject it. This diversion can occur by cannulation of either the atria or the ventricles. These illustrations show some of the cannulation options.

There are three types of VAD placement:

• A right ventricular assist device (RVAD) provides pulmonary support by diverting blood from the right atrium or failing right ventricle to the VAD, which then pumps the blood to the pulmonary circulation via the VAD connection to the left pulmonary artery. If a patient needs right-sided support for a failing right ventricle and is also having oxygenation issues, there is an option of adding an oxygenator to the RVAD. (See the below illustration.)

LVAD

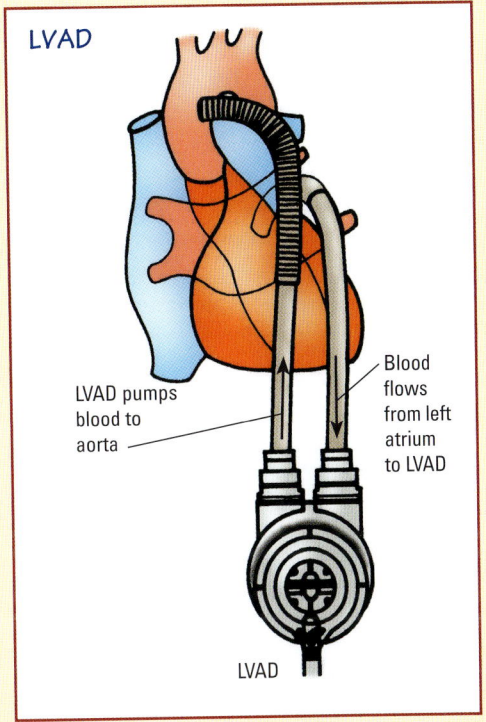

LVAD pumps blood to aorta

Blood flows from left atrium to LVAD

LVAD

RVAD

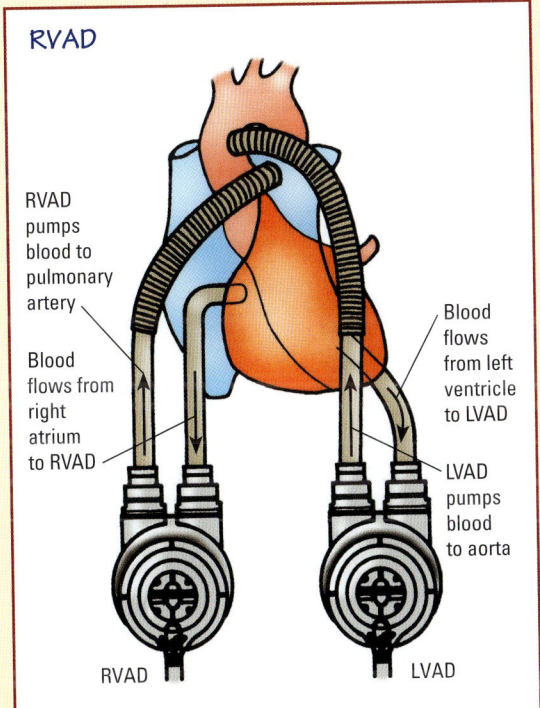

RVAD pumps blood to pulmonary artery

Blood flows from right atrium to RVAD

Blood flows from left ventricle to LVAD

LVAD pumps blood to aorta

RVAD   LVAD

BiVAD

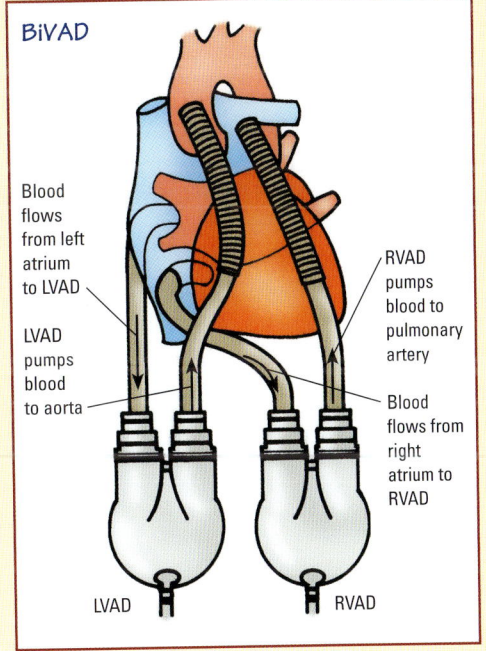

Blood flows from left atrium to LVAD

LVAD pumps blood to aorta

RVAD pumps blood to pulmonary artery

Blood flows from right atrium to RVAD

LVAD   RVAD

• With a left ventricular assist device (LVAD), blood flows from the left atrium or ventricle to the VAD, which then pumps blood back to the body via the VAD connection to the aorta. (See the top right illustration in this box.)

• When an RVAD and an LVAD are both used, it is referred to as *biventricular (BiVAD) support*. (See the illustration at right.)

Potential complications

Despite the use of anticoagulants, the VAD may cause thrombi formation, leading to pulmonary embolism or stroke. Thrombi that form inside of the VAD itself can cause the VAD to no longer function for the patient. That patient may require the use of medications to break up the clot, or in the worst-case scenario, a pump exchange. The biggest reason for a patient with a VAD to be readmitted to the hospital is gastrointestinal bleeding. When patients are on either anticoagulant or antiplatelet therapy, arterial malformations may occur predominantly in the gastrointestinal tract. Immediate postoperative complications may include acute right ventricle (RV) failure, cardiac tamponade, and bleeding. Patients can also develop late RV failure. Other possible complications include heart failure, bleeding, cardiac tamponade, or infection.

Clinical assessment

Care and assessment of patients with VADs require special attention. Equipment operation must be assessed, and because patients are often discharged to home, patient education about use and care is essential. Patients will also need to be instructed about their activities of daily living such as no bathing or submersion in water (however, showering is usually allowed); and care of their exit site and driveline (percutaneous lead that exits the body and connects to equipment), with scheduled sterile dressing changes and adherence to medical therapies, such as medications, labwork, and follow-up provider visits. Information about what to do in an emergency must be part of their education.

Monitoring blood pressure in CF LVADs can be a challenge; normal systolic and diastolic sounds may not be heard, and often the mean arterial pressure (mAP) is monitored. For example, patients with CF LVADs may need to keep their mAPs within a certain range (recommended 75 to 85 mm Hg). Most VADs require that patients' blood be anticoagulated, so the administration of anticoagulants and antiplatelets is critical, as well as monitoring their effect (i.e., international normalized ratio [INR] values). As opposed to pre-VAD implant fluid restrictions, patients with a VAD need to maintain adequate volume status and be well hydrated. Lastly, monitoring for complications such as infection, bleeding, thrombosis, and device malfunction must be understood and communicated to the health care team. All VAD centers have a 24-hour emergency line that their patients are instructed to call with any issues they are having related to the VAD.

Quick quiz

Show and tell

Identify the assessment technique being used in each illustration.

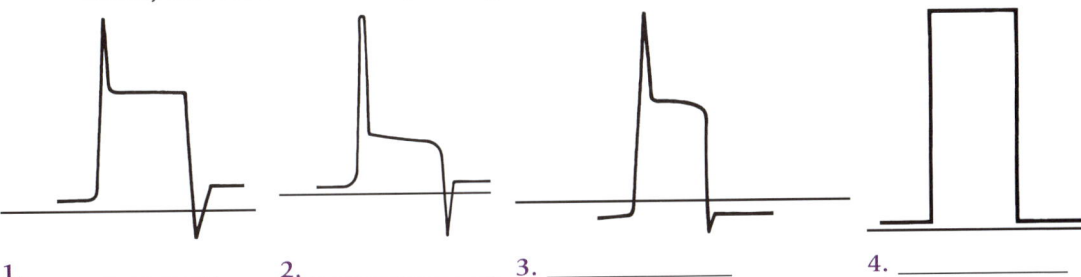

1. _____

2. _____

3. _____

4. _____

True or false

Indicate whether each statement is true or false.

1. VADs can be pulsatile or continuous flow.

   _____

2. Patients with VADs can go swimming.

   _____

3. A VAD that supports the left ventricle is called an LVAD.

   _____

4. VADs are only used as a bridge to transplant.

   _____

Multiple response

1. What is monitored in patients with a VAD? (Check all that apply.)
   A. blood pressure or mAP
   B. anticoagulation status
   C. signs/symptoms of infection
   D. understanding of VAD equipment and care
   E. volume or hydration status

Answers: Show and tell: 1. balloon pressure baseline elevation; 2. low balloon pressure plateau; 3. balloon pressure depression; 4. high balloon pressure plateau. *True or false:* 1. True, 2. False, 3. True, 4. False. *Multiple response:* All choices are correct.

Selected references

Chemielinski, A., & Koons, B. (2017). Nursing care for the patient with a left ventricular assist device. *Nursing, 20*(5), 34–40. https://doi.org/10.1097/01.NURSE.0000515503.80037.07

Delgado, S. (2023). *AACN essentials of critical care nursing* (5th ed.). McGraw-Hill.

Glazier, J., & Kaki, A. (2019). The Impella device: Historical background, clinical applications and future directions. *International Journal of Angiography, 28*(2), 118–123. https://doi.org/10.1055/s-0038-1676369

Johnson, K. (2023). *AACN procedure manual for high acuity, progressive and critical care* (8th ed.). Elsevier.

Lippincott, Williams and Wilkins. (2022). Lippincott nursing procedures (9th ed.). Author.

McLaughlin, M. A. (2025). *Cardiovascular care made incredibly easy* (5th ed.). Wolters Kluwer.

Morton, P. G., & Thurman, P. (2024). *Critical care nursing: A holistic approach* (12th ed.). Lippincott Williams & Wilkins.

Perpetua, E., & Keegan, P. (2021). *Cardiac nursing* (7th ed.). Lippincott Williams & Wilkins.

Index

QUADM0924